Developing Norm-Referenced Standardized Tests

Developing Norm-Referenced Standardized Tests

Lucy Jane Miller
Editor

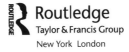
Routledge
Taylor & Francis Group
New York London

First published 1989 by The Haworth Press, Inc.

Published 2019 by Routledge
52 Vanderbilt Avenue, New York, NY 10017
2 Park Square, Milton Park, Abingdon, Oxon OX14 4RN

Routledge is an imprint of the Taylor & Francis Group, an informa business

Developing Norm-Referenced Standardized Tests has also been published as *Physical & Occupational Therapy in Pediatrics*, Volume 9, Number 1 1989.

Library of Congress Cataloging-in-Publication Data

Developing norm-referenced standardized tests / Lucy Jane Miller, editor.
    p. cm.
    "Also . . . published as Physical & occupational therapy in pediatrics, volume 9, number 1, 1989" – T.p. verso.
    Bibliography: p.
    ISBN 0-86656-883-2
    1. Occupational therapy – Research – Methodology. 2. Physical therapy – Research – Methodology. 3. Norm-referenced tests. I. Miller, Lucy J.
RM735.42.D38 1989
615.8'515 – dc19   88-36502
                                 CIP

ISBN 13: 978-0-86656-883-8 (hbk)

Dedicated to the memory of
A. Jean Ayres

July 18, 1920 — December 16, 1988

Who took brilliant clinical insights and embodied them in a standarized format, defining them with self-imposed scientific discipline;

Who struggled to create and maintain a place within her chosen profession in which her work could flourish;

Who ultimately created a space for the rest of us where new and innovative ideas could grow within a supportive climate of excitement and scientific inquiry.

Developing Norm-Referenced Standardized Tests

CONTENTS

Foreword xi
A. Jean Ayres

Preface xiii
Jerry A. Johnson

Acknowledgements xix

**Chapter 1: Measurement in Developmental Therapy:
Past, Present, and Future** 1
Suzann K. Campbell

Introduction 1
History of Standardized Testing 2
Lack of Testing Instruments 5
Rationale for Increased Use of Standardized Tests 8
The Priority to Develop Validated Tools 9
Summary and Recommendations 10

Chapter 2: Planning the Initial Version 15
Bette R. Bonder

Introduction 15
Formulating the Idea 16
Reviewing the Literature 19
Identification of Specific Content for Items 20
The Table of Specifications 21
Item Format 22
Item Development 28
Planning the Standardization Process 32
Statistical Consultation 32

Ethical Considerations   33
Funding the Plan   37
Summary and Recommendations   39

**Chapter 3: Designing and Implementing Research
    on the Development Editions of the Test   43**
       Jan Gwyer

Introduction   43
Purpose for Conducting a Development Edition   45
Selecting the Development Edition Sample   46
Test Administration Procedures   47
Analysis of Item Characteristics   52
Evaluating Reliability and Validity   56
Summary and Recommendations   59

Chapter 4: Standardizing an Assessment   63
       James Gyurke
       Aurelio Prifitera

Introduction   63
Developing the Timeline and Budget   64
Examiner Recruitment and Training   69
Selecting a Sample   70
Bias Review   77
Data Collection   78
Data Analysis   80
Reliability and Validity   85
Norms Development   86
Publication   86
Summary and Recommendations   87

Chapter 5: Norms and Scores   91
       Sharon Cermak

Introduction   91
Statistical Concepts   92
Norms and Scores   98
Summary and Recommendations   113

Chapter 6: Reliability 125
Jean C. Deitz

Introduction 125
Types of Reliability 126
Designing Reliability Research for a Test 135
Statistics 137
Summary and Recommendations 144

Chapter 7: Validity 149
Winnie W. Dunn

Introduction 149
Validity in Therapeutic Practice 150
Basic Issues in Validity Research 151
Types of Validity Studies 153
Summary and Recommendations 164

Chapter 8: Preparing the Examiner's Manual 169
Tracy A. Sprong

Introduction 169
Preliminary Preparation 170
Getting Started 171
The Drafting Process 172
Final Organization 175
Summary and Recommendations 179

Epilogue: Test Development on the Installment Plan
***or* "How I Developed a Test in 27,000 Easy Steps"** 185
Lucy Jane Miller

Appendixes 195

ABOUT THE EDITOR

Lucy Jane Miller, PhD, OTR, Executive Director, The Foundation for Knowledge in Development, Englewood, Colorado, has been actively involved in early childhood research and test development for over 15 years. She is most widely recognized as the author of the Miller Assessment for Preschoolers (MAP), a nationally standardized, norm-referenced test. She is currently involved in two test development projects, one to develop a short developmental screening for preschoolers and the other to develop an assessment for infants and toddlers. Her research experience includes the standardization of the MAP and subsequent longitudinal predictive validity research, both large-scale national studies.

Dr. Miller holds a doctorate in early childhood special education, has published numerous technical and review papers, and was recently named a Charter Member to the American Occupational Therapy Foundation Academy of Research.

Foreword

In the long run, men hit only what they aim at. Therefore, though they should fail immediately, they had better aim at something high.

— Thoreau
"Economy" Walden *(1854)*

This collection of papers signals the early years of an important era, especially in occupational therapy. It reflects an attitude of professional and scientific responsibility that has been slow in coming but is now well on its way. A science is marked by the quality of and degree to which it measures the parameters of its field. Measuring instruments are critical tools for acquiring knowledge and it is difficult to acquire knowledge without them. The more precisely behavior is measured the better it is understood.

Tests yield numbers and numbers can do things that words or ideas cannot do. In occupational and physical therapy measurement is central to differential diagnosis, gain or loss assessment, establishing client status, predicting response to therapy, building and testing theory, and conveying information across fields. It is difficult to accomplish any of these goals without some form of measurement.

Recognition and acceptance of the need for measuring instruments is only the first step; the method of actual development of a test is described by this issue. The therapy fields face testing problems rather specific to themselves. Procedures that yield the most clinically meaningful information sometimes yield the least attractive statistical analysis. Therapists often measure functions that are

---

A. Jean Ayres, PhD, OTR, developed the *Sensory Integration and Praxis Test* and the *Southern California Sensory Integration Tests*. She is Emeritus member of the Board of Directors, Center for Study of Sensory Integrative Dysfunction, 5339 Bindewald Rd., Torrance, CA 90505.

not naturally distributed according to the Gausian model on which most statistical methods in the behavioral sciences are based. Sometimes a linear transformation of raw scores into a different metric system is sufficient to meet the problem, but sometimes it is not. Occupational and physical therapists usually evaluate individuals whose performance falls below age expectations, yet most statistical procedures and expectations are based on a "normal" population.

Most importantly, the well-established behavioral sciences expect a quality of instrumentation the development of which requires large monetary expenditures, services of specialists in measurement, and cooperation on the part of many therapists. Meeting those expectations is often unrealistic, necessitating contentment with a more gradual course of development in which a test is designed, used, analyzed, and re-designed many times over many years in the clinical situation. It is a wise test-building method, for the design of a test is its most important attribute. When a test has proven its worth, it is then ready for a larger investment. The important thing is to measure the best way possible in a given situation. This volume will help accomplish that purpose.

A. Jean Ayres

Preface

The great tragedy of science — the slaying of a beautiful hypothesis by an ugly fact.

— Thomas Henry Huxley (1825-1895)
"Biogenesis and Abiogenesis"

Developing Norm-Referenced Standardized Tests, the title and theme of this special collection, has particular relevance for occupational and physical therapists. Its purpose is to provide a "how-to" manual for use by therapists who want to construct a *norm-referenced test*. In essence, this work will describe the process of developing standardized norm-referenced tests.

Members of both the occupational and physical therapy professions have increasingly engaged in the process of expanding and revising theories which undergird the practice of each profession, primarily by testing the hypotheses associated with specific theories. Clinicians in both professions also seek to develop tests that will enable them to (1) more precisely define the problems with which they are concerned and (2) select treatment procedures that will produce the most effective treatment outcomes.

The development of instrumentation enables the theoretician/scientist/clinician to describe and measure certain phenomena which are of interest and is a crucial component of knowledge development and scientific exploration and growth. In professions which are and have been practice-oriented since their founding, clinicians, as well as theoreticians and researchers, must develop an under-

Jerry A. Johnson, EdD, OTR, FAOTA, is President of Context, Inc., P.O. Box 6885, Denver, CO 80206. Formerly, she served as President of the American Occupational Therapy Association and as Professor of Occupational Therapy at Boston University and the Washington University in St. Louis.

standing of the importance of research and its potential contributions to the improvement of their practice.

Two types of tests, *norm-referenced tests* and *criterion-referenced tests*, are relevant for the clinician who is beginning research. A norm-referenced test is one in which an individual's performance is compared against the performance of other individuals (a referent or normative group). Most common among this type of tests are intelligence or aptitude tests such as the *Bayley Scales of Infant Development*,[1] *Wechsler Intelligence Scale for Children-Revised*,[2] and the *McCarthy Scales of Children's Abilities*.[3]

A criterion-referenced test compares an individual's performance to a predetermined behavioral criterion or content domain.[4] Criterion-referenced tests are used primarily in education, and include tests assessing basic mastery of skills, such as the *Metropolitan Achievement Test, Sixth Edition*,[5] and the *Criterion-Referenced Curriculum-Mathematics*.[6] In the therapies there are several criterion-referenced checklists such as the *Developmental Programming for Infants and Young Children*[7] and the *Vulpe Assessment Battery*.[8] A criterion-referenced test indicates whether or not the individual has learned certain skills and may describe which skills are learned.

In summary, a criterion-referenced test reports the examinee's performance in terms of what s/he knows and can do, whereas the norm-referenced test reports how the examinee's performance compares to the performance of others. One other difference in these two types of tests is that norm-referenced tests tend to be standardized, whereas criterion-referenced tests are not necessarily standardized.[9] While the content of this volume only discusses *norm-referenced tests*, both types of tests are important but in different ways. Table 1 describes the differences between norm-referenced tests and criterion-referenced tests.

This special collection is designed for therapists who have an interest in conducting research, either collaboratively with established scientists or independently, to pursue questions of interest. More specifically, the content of this issue will take the reader through a step-by-step process, including identification of a concept that should be subjected to testing, development of appropriate test items, and the procedures for standardizing a norm-referenced test.

In Chapter 1, the reader is introduced to the historical perspective

Table 1. Differences Between Norm-Referenced Tests and Criterion-Referenced Tests.

	Norm-Referenced Tests	Criterion-Referenced Tests
Purpose	Comparison among examinees	Examinee performance in relation to set of competencies
Content Specificity	• More general content • Often greater breadth of coverage	• More detailed content specifications • May use behavioral or instructional objectives
Test Development	• Use of item statistics (difficulty and discrimination indexes) serve in item selection. • Select moderate difficulty items and high discrimination.	Content includes items passed or failed by nearly all examinees.
Test Score Generalizability	• Generally do not make generalizations from norm-referenced achievement test scores.	Generalize performance to larger domains of content defining the competencies.

Table by Sharon Cermak, EdD, OTR

of and projected trends associated with test development. The rationale of standardized testing is discussed, as is the need for involvement of occupational and physical therapists in test development.

Chapter 2 assists the reader in the formulation of ideas leading to construction of an appropriate test. The components of planning the development process are elaborated, from the review of the theoretical and research literature to the resources available to fund stages of the research.

In Chapter 3, the importance and step-by-step details of the Development Edition phase are illuminated. During this stage, administration procedures are clarified and item analysis is conducted to determine whether the items have good psychometric characteristics. A large item pool is generated and studied extensively to determine which items should be selected for large scale standardization.

Procedures for standardization of the test, including development of a scoring system and testing for reliability and validity, are discussed in Chapter 4, 5, 6, and 7. Chapter 8 outlines methods of preparing an examiner's manual and presentation of its content. A "personal note" from the editor of this special collection is also included in which she recounts experiences as a test developer.

Standardization of tests in a profession forms the foundation for its credibility and begins to delineate the parameters of practice and expertise which clinicians, educators, and/or researchers in other disciplines can expect of its members. In effect, practice based on results and information obtained from standardized tests developed for specific purposes establishes a profession's claim to certain areas of knowledge, practice, and responsibility. It moves the profession's practice from a "belief" system to a foundation which others can evaluate objectively.

The authors of this issue are making a significant contribution to the continuing development of knowledge and research in both occupational and physical therapy. Not only will this increase understanding of the process of test development for instruments which are already available, but it is intended to stimulate the development of new instrumentation by providing a step-by-step guide for those interested in developing a new test. Developing more standardized tests in the therapies will contribute to the continuing intellectual growth of members of these two professions, and to greater public recognition and acceptance of their theoretical foundations and therapeutic procedures.

This work is timely and is recommended for study by all occupational and physical therapists who want to actively participate in the challenges that confront their respective professions and who desire to pursue their own professional growth.

Jerry A. Johnson

REFERENCES

1. Bayley N: *Bayley Scales of Infant Development*. New York, Psychological Corporation, 1969.

2. Wechsler D: *Wechsler Intelligence Scale for Children-Revised*. New York, Psychological Corporation, 1974.

3. McCarthy D: *McCarthy Scales of Children's Abilities*. New York, Psychological Corporation, 1972.

4. Anastasi A: *Psychological Testing*, ed 6. New York, Collier Macmillan Publishers, 1988.

5. Farr R, Prescott G, Balow I, Hogan T: *Metropolitan Achievement Tests, Sixth Edition-Reading Diagnostic Tests*. New York, Psychological Corporation, 1987.

6. Stephens T: *Criterion-Referenced Curriculum-Mathematics*. New York, Psychological Corporation, 1982.

7. Rogers SJ, D'Eugenio DB, Moersch M: *Developmental Programming for Infants and Young Children*. Ann Arbor, MI, University of Michigan Press, 1977.

8. Vulpe SG: *Vulpe Assessment Battery*, ed 2. Toronto, National Institute on Mental Retardation, 1977.

9. Goodwin WL, Driscoll L: *Handbook for Measurement and Evaluation in Early Childhood Education*. San Francisco, Jossey-Bass Publishers, 1980.

Acknowledgments

The editor sincerely appreciates the flexibility of all the authors for allowing segments of their manuscripts to be used in other chapters. The overall continuity of this work was enhanced greatly. With a complex subject such as test development, many aspects of the process overlap. It follows that the contributing authors, writing independently, also overlapped in content. To avoid possible redundancy for the reader, sections from some chapters were integrated into others. This work represents a collaborative effort by all the authors who generously provided their time and expertise. The editor would like to specifically acknowledge the following contributions:

Sharon Cermak: discussion and table about criterion-referenced tests in the Foreword.

Winnie Dunn: discussions of operationalizing constructs in Chapter 1; operational definitions, table of specifications, and item selection in Chapter 2; and testing conditions in Chapter 3.

James Gyurke and Aurelio Prifitera: discussion of criterion-referenced tests in the Foreword.

Susan Kaplan: providing discussion and illustrations of the normal curve and positive and negative skew for Chapter 5.

Tracy Sprong: discussion of ethical considerations in Chapter 2.

Also special thanks are extended to Richard T. Campbell, PhD, Peter Schouten, MS, and Gale Roid, PhD, for their statistical consultation and editorial assistance, and to Debbie Campbell for journal reference checking.

Chapter 1

Measurement in Developmental Therapy: Past, Present, and Future

Suzann K. Campbell

People seldom learn from the mistakes of others — not because they deny the value of the past, but because they are faced with new problems.

> — *Ilya Ehrenburg*
> *"What I Have Learned"*
> Saturday Review, *September 30, 1967*

INTRODUCTION

Physical and occupational therapists recently have generated a flurry of activity aimed at development of new standardized assessment tools for use in pediatric clinical and educational settings. For example, the *Miller Assessment for Preschoolers*,[1] the *Movement Assessment of Infants*,[2] and the *Hughes Gross Motor Assessment*[3] are therapist-designed test that have become available in the past decade. Nevertheless, the subdisciplines of pediatric occupational and physical therapy have not yet embraced wholeheartedly the concept that therapists routinely should use and develop their own standardized assessments. Nor have professionals in these fields put

Suzann K. Campbell, PT, PhD, FAPTA, is Professor of Physical Therapy at the College of Associated Health Professions at the University of Illinois at Chicago, 1919 W. Taylor St., Chicago, IL 60612.

While writing this paper, the author was partially supported by Grant MCJ 9101 from the Bureau of Health Care Delivery and Assistance, USPHS.

1

those tests that are available to work in improving clinical diagnostic capabilities and accountability to clients and the public for the costly treatment provided.

The purpose of this introductory chapter is to describe the history of standardized testing, the current problem of lack of testing instruments, and the rationale for increased use of standardized tests in developmental therapy settings. The need for pediatric occupational and physical therapists to develop more scientifically validated tools is also addressed.

HISTORY OF STANDARDIZED TESTING

Critical to the future development of occupational and physical therapy as scientific and clinical disciplines is the generation of measurement tools specific to client needs. Many clinicians are depending upon tests developed by psychologists and other professionals with different types of clients or goals in mind. Worse, a trend of the 1970s in some areas of the subdisciplines was to avoid formal testing.

According to Nunnally, the movement toward standardized testing was generated in the last century by Darwin's theory of evolution.[4] The concept of "survival of the fittest" led to interest in measuring individual differences in abilities of various types. Galton, the founder of the eugenics movement aimed at improving the human race, studied the heritability of human traits using tests of sensory discrimination. Sensory acuity was believed to be the basis of intellect. Interest was so great that people were willing to pay for the opportunity to be measured with Galton's techniques! His contributions were important for their explicit recognition of (1) the need for standardization in testing—the concept that each individual should be tested with the same items under the same conditions and with standard instructions, (2) for emphasizing the importance of individual differences in abilities, and (3) for the development of correlational methods, later refined by Pearson, with which to analyze the collected data.

Binet and Simon developed the first test of global intelligence in 1905 at the behest of the French government which had recognized the need for developing a testing tool to evaluate and classify children who were too mentally deficient to profit from schooling.[4] This work led to the concept of norms for performance of children at different ages, calculation of mental ages, and eventually the search for factors in human intelligence. Psychologists, such as Spearman and Thurstone, theorized that intelligence included a general factor, g, and specific factors, such as verbal, numerical, spatial, memory, reasoning, analogy, and perceptual abilities. They developed factor analysis as a methodological approach to studying human cognitive abilities. Piaget further advanced the study of cognitive performance by carefully studying the processes, rather than the content, of mental development. This produced a revolutionary and continuing impact on developmental psychology.

The standardized testing movement spread widely to include assessment of most areas of human ability, and made significant contributions in practical application to personnel selection, school admissions, and psychiatric and other medical diagnostic tasks.[4] Rare is the person who has never taken a standardized test of some kind before reaching adolescence. Although standardized tests are continually criticized for labeling and lack of cultural validity for some groups in the population, such as minorities, they remain the best known means of sorting, classifying, diagnosing, and measuring progress.

Researchers have also studied the factors contributing to motor development, to motor learning, and to skilled motor performance. Developmental therapists have been interested in studying the relationships between motor milestones, developmental reflexes and reactions, and "quality" of movement. Though interested, little advancement has been made in the measurement of motor dysfunction or progress during therapy. Undoubtedly, progress has been slow in part because of the tremendous complexity involved in sorting out the many factors, both sensory and motor, that contribute to skilled motor performance. "Quality" of movement is difficult to capture and describe because it does not consist of a single factor, but rather is a jargon term inclusive of coordination, postural control, and balance.[5]

Research on motor development has resulted in the identification of nine different aspects of gross and fine motor development in normal children from preschool age to adolescence.[6] Specific factors implicated in gross motor abilities were speed, static and dynamic body balance, coordination, and strength. For fine motor performance, the identified factors were visual-motor tracking, response speed to a visual stimulus, visual-motor control of the hand, and upper extremity speed and precision in manipulation. Taken together, these factors were believed to include the elements of speed, precision, strength, balance, and coordination.

These factors unquestionably are important in motor performance of children with developmental disabilities as well. The abnormal sensorimotor system, however, presents a more complex measurement problem. For example, researchers have not yet been able to identify and isolate the specific factors operating on motor performance in the various types of central nervous system (CNS) dysfunction. A review of the literature on motor control deficits in children and adults with cerebral palsy (CP), however, suggests that alterations in limb stiffness, reflex gain, sensory receptive fields, and movement synergies are candidates as factors in addition to those involved in normal motor performance.[5,7-13] Finally, research in motor learning suggests that likely factors important in both normal and pathologic movement include repetition, knowledge of results, motor memory, perceptual factors, specificity of exercise relative to movement goals, and the environmental context.[14]

Occupational and physical therapists historically have been slow to develop and standardize tests for use in studying motor development, control, and learning, and for diagnosing problems or measuring progress in clients. As an example, in the area of motor development in children with cerebral palsy, several tests appeared in the 1950s and 1960s. They were based primarily on the Gesell motor milestones, but added special tests of speed or ability to perform activities involving rhythmic reversal of direction.[15,16] These tests were aimed at quantifying motor performance in children with CP in a way that would produce developmental quotients or motor ages. Several important papers also were published which emphasized the importance of assessing and documenting motor development in quantitative ways that would reliably capture the progress of handicapped children.[17,18] Nonetheless, a statement made in 1951 that "We are unable to describe the patient with cerebral palsy in any way which lends itself to a statistical analysis"[15,p.698] remains true today.

The next decade produced almost no work on measurement of motor performance in CP other than gait analyses for assessment of outcome of orthopedic procedures[13,19-20] and a few tests of specific functions. The 1980s saw the introduction of several new research tools for the study of pathokinesiology[7,21-23] and introduction of the *Movement Assessment of Infants*,[2] a promising new tool still under development, but limited to neurologic assessment in infancy.

Professionals in occupational therapy have accomplished more than those in physical therapy in developing tools for assessing children with mild neurologic dysfunction, such as the *Sensory Integration and Praxis Test*[24] and the *Miller Assessment for Preschoolers*.[1] Yet much remains to be done.

LACK OF TESTING INSTRUMENTS

Important questions arise when examining the current lack of testing instruments. Why are there no universally agreed upon assessment batteries for each type of pediatric developmental disability? Why are formal tests necessary to supplement the clinician's observational skills? What are the consequences of this lack of objective measurement tools?

No Universally Agreed Upon Assessment Batteries

Six main reasons surface in response to the issue of no universally agreed upon assessment batteries. First, cerebral palsy and other developmental disabilities are complex and those children afflicted are difficult to study scientifically. Second, the professions of occupational and physical therapy are service-oriented. Third, many academics are isolated from the clinical setting, and therefore, from joint research with clinicians. Fourth, historically faculty members have had high teaching loads, a lack of research training and experience, and a low level of psychometric knowledge. Fifth, funding for large scale research and development is difficult to obtain in fields which do not have a history of excellence in this area. And finally, much of the neurodevelopmental (NDT) and Rood clinical establishment embody anti-quantification, anti-scientific characteristics.

Clinical leaders in the area of neurodevelopment have contributed significantly to developing the theory and to teaching the art of clinical practice while advancing *scientific* clinical practice hardly at all. Although the sensory integration community has made significant contributions toward establishing valid and reliable measurement practices, much more remains to be accomplished. In their thirst for better tools, clinicians have either used ill-suited tests from other disciplines, such as psychology, or even more frequently uniformly rejected other available tests because of their weaknesses in accomplishing what they were never intended to do. Instead, many clinicians have created their own so-called "tests" of highly questionable reliability and validity.

Necessity of Formal Tests to Supplement Observational Skills

A long list of references can be found in the literature to document the notorious unreliability of the clinician's diagnostic capabilities. Sackett and colleagues described a number of studies documenting the serious consequences of clinical misjudgment.[25] In one study of 93 adolescents who previously had been labeled as having organic heart disease or rheumatic fever, reevaluation revealed that 81 percent of the children studied actually had normal hearts.[26] Of special interest to occupational and physical therapists is that the misdiagnosed children experienced restriction of physical and social activity as much as the children with true heart disease; 30 (40 percent) of the 75 children with no current heart disease were restricted in some way.

Articles published recently in the professional literature of physical therapy have noted problems with the reliability of observational gait analysis,[27] an infant motor performance scale,[28] and goniometry.[29,30] Sources of error in clinician assessments include the examiner, the exam in use, and the inherent variability of human subjects.[25] For example, clinician judgments vary because of biologic variation from time to time in sensory acuity, variation in application of diagnostic criteria to clinical evidence, bias in expectations, errors of omission or commission in gathering evidence, and the tendency to record inference rather than evidence. Clients, too (especially children!), vary across assessments, may be influenced by medications or illness, and have varying capabilities to respond to questions or perform on demand. The examination situation itself may also contribute to unreliability in judgments. The busy outpatient clinic is not conducive to careful evaluation of child development, therapist-client communication may break down, and diagnostic equipment may malfunction.

It has become a maxim of clinical decision-making theory that to advance the art and science of clinical practice, the tool that must be improved is the clinician. Other suggestions for improving clinical judgments include: establishing an appropriate environment for evaluation, reliability training with colleagues, seeking corroboration of key clinical findings by repetition, blind evaluations of clients by colleagues, and using quantitative tools, such as standardized tests, to verify and document clinical observational findings.[25]

Consequences of the Lack of Measurement Tools

Mere need to increase the use of standardized tests, however, is not the total solution to the problem. In 1976, Lewko vividly illustrated the dimensions of the problem of poor use of testing tools in pediatric therapy.[31] The researcher surveyed dozens of pediatric institutions to discover what tests were used to assess motor development, whether they were used for appropriate purposes, and how informed users were about the information provided in test manuals. Respondents (largely occupational or physical therapists) reported poor knowledge of information sources about motor development tests, inappropriate use of standardized tests, and considerable use of therapist-designed tests that were not standardized or examined for reliability and validity. At best, this represents poor service to clients. At worst, it represents unethical practice that may produce considerable harm by resultant mislabeling, expensive provision of unnecessary services, or failure to identify and treat problems amenable to developmental therapy. Such practices also hinder the development of a scientific body of knowledge on which to base advancement of clinical practice.

RATIONALE FOR INCREASED USE OF STANDARDIZED TESTS

The importance of using and developing standardized measures for assessment of clients and documentation of progress under treatment can perhaps best be described by considering the alternatives.[4] Without them, we must base our clinical practice on subjective, personal judgments prone to each of the errors mentioned previously. Their major advantages are objectivity, quantitative scores, contribution to communication among professionals, and, although expensive to develop initially, their cost/benefit ratio in application to practice. Finally, without the ability to quantify variables of importance to clinical practice through use of standardized measures, the scientific inquiry process cannot progress to advance the field through research. It is an axiom in science that progress in any field is often tied to the development of new measuring tools. The use of these tools allows the revelation of previously unknown facts and drives theory, practice, and new research, often explosively.

In the area of pediatrics, one need think only of the *Brazelton Neonatal Behavioral Assessment Scale* to identify the potentialities involved in the development of new tools for use in practice and research.[32] Appearance of this scale generated an explosion of research on the interactive characteristics of neonatal personality, applied research on individual differences, and on the influence of environmental exposure to drugs, intervention, premature birth and other factors. The scale has also led to new tools for assessing premature and other high risk infants, opening up still more avenues for clinical practice and research.

On the other hand, failure of occupational and physical therapy to develop tools for measuring the elusive property of motor performance, "quality" of movement, results in highly subjective and individualized interpretation. The absence of statistical analysis or "numbers" to define motor performance creates an inability to communicate what it is to other professionals or even to each other and requires the use of costly anecdotal records to document patient progress. Only scientific studies can validate the importance of the qualitative aspects of motor performance, its amenability to treatment, its diagnostic value, or, indeed, *whether it even exists as a real phenomenon.*

THE PRIORITY TO DEVELOP VALIDATED TOOLS

As professional disciplines committed to scientific clinical practice and to provision of the best possible services to clients, available measurement tools must be used appropriately. Also, attention must be devoted to development of unique tests for assessing motor performance, occupational behavior, and functional capacities; for diagnosing those aspects of developmental disabilities that are amenable to therapeutic intervention; and for documenting progress and predicting to ultimate outcome of therapy.

Current Trends

Current trends suggest that these goals will be achieved. Already, the increase in numbers of therapists pursuing advanced degrees has had an impact on the professional community as these individuals have been exposed to education in measurement and scientific approaches to clinical practice. Therapists are coming to understand that if the validity of their instrumentation is questioned, so, too, will be the validity of their intervention. To the credit of the professions, therapists are becoming increasingly interested in use of standardized tests and have more knowledge concerning measurement theory and concepts than ever before. Lewko's study should be replicated in an attempt to assess whether this new knowledge and interest has already resulted in improved test usage.[31]

The advent of new tests and the power they convey are also having an important impact on pediatric occupational and physical therapy and will generate the desire for more such tools. External pressures for accountability, cost control, and cost/benefit analyses, and pressures from physicians and others to document efficacy are forcing change on these professions that can only lead to increased efforts to measure sensorimotor performance in scientifically defensible ways. Although no test has ever been designed without error, the day is at hand when the parameters of developmental motor performance can be isolated and quantified. This will lead to improvements in the diagnosis of sensorimotor disabilities amenable to treatment with occupational or physical therapy, the development of new treatment strategies that are more specific and efficacious, and the documentation of the cost-effective benefits of intervention.

These trends will also lead to the development of a scientific body of knowledge in each of these fields that will provide important support for upgrading education and practice, engender financial resources for research, and raise their status in the health care and education fields. Communication with specialists in education, medicine, and psychology, as well as those in other health care professions, will be improved. The increase in scientific documentation will enhance the status of occupational and physical therapists and their work.

SUMMARY AND RECOMMENDATIONS

In occupational and physical therapy, many constructs have not been previously operationalized or measured. Therefore, many opportunities exist to make significant and useful contributions to knowledge about human performance. This condition reflects these disciplines' unique historical development. In some ways the current developmental status of occupational and physical therapy is similar to the field of psychology prior to the time of immense growth in tests and measurements.

It is important for therapists to recognize that both clinicians and researchers can, and must, contribute to this enterprise. Scientists with clinical and psychometric knowledge are needed to plan, develop, validate, and publish new testing instruments. Educators are needed to teach measurement principles and critical analysis of the clinical literature at every level of the educational ladder. Both scientists and educators are needed to serve on grant review panels that fund the needed research, and, along with clinicians, to sit on task forces and committees that establish standards for scientific clinical practice. Clinicians are the major source of data on problems that need to be solved, tests that must be developed, and, of critical importance, of patients that must be used during the test development, norming, and validation process. Only with everyone working together can the job be accomplished.

A final crucial ingredient is *support* for the enterprise from the total community of interest — mutual acceptance of initial, less than perfect efforts that begin the process; sharing of data, patients, and technical support; and acknowledgment that continual, gradual improvement based on critical analysis of results is necessary to keep the process alive and productive. To these ends, this work is devoted to raising the consciousness of developmental therapists regarding the value of norm-referenced standardized tests and aiding the scientific and clinical communities of interest in gaining the knowledge and skills necessary to develop the tools needed for the next century.

REFERENCES

1. Miller LJ: *Miller Assessment for Preschoolers*. San Antonio, TX, Psychological Corporation, 1988, 1982.

2. Chandler L, Andrews M, Swanson M: *Movement Assessment of Infants*. Rolling Bay, WA, Infant Movement Research, 1980.

3. Hughes JE: *Manual for the Hughes Basic Gross Motor Assessment*. Goldon, CO, Jeanne E. Hughes, 1979.

4. Nunnally JC: *Psychometric Theory*, ed 2. New York, McGraw Hill, 1978.

5. Campbell SK: Assessment of the child with CNS dysfunction, in Rothstein JM (ed): *Measurement in Physical Therapy*. New York, Churchill Livingstone, 1985, pp 207-228.

6. Krus PH, Bruininks RH, Robertson G: Structure of motor abilities in children: *Percept Mot Skills* 52: 119-129, 1981.

7. Barolot-Romana G, Davis R: Neurophysiological mechanisms in abnormal reflex activities in cerebral palsy and spinal spasticity. *J Neurol Neuosurg Psychiat* 43: 333-342, 1980.

8. Berger W, Quintern J, Dietz V: Stance and gait perturbations in children: Developmental aspects of compensatory mechanisms. *Electroencephalogra Clin Neurophysiol* 61: 385-395, 1985.

9. Campbell SK: Central nervous system dysfunction in children, in Campbell SK (ed): *Pediatric Neurologic Physical Therapy*. New York, Churchill Livingstone, 1984, pp 1-12.

10. Milner-Brown HS, Penn RD: Pathophysiological mechanisms in cerebral palsy. *J Neurol Neurosurg Psychiatr* 42: 606-618, 1979.

11. Nashner LM, Shumway-Cook A, Marin O: Stance posture control in se-

lect groups of children with cerebral palsy: Deficits in sensory organization and muscular coordination. *Exp Brain Res* 49: 393-409, 1983.

12. Neilson PD: Voluntary control of arm movement in athetotic patients. *J Neurol Neurosurg Psychiatr* 37: 162-170, 1974.

13. Perry J, Hoffer MM: Preoperative and postoperative dynamic electromyography as an aid in planning tendon transfers in children with cerebral palsy. *J Bone Joint Surg* 59-A: 531-537, 1977.

14. Kelso, JAS: *Human Motor Behavior—An Introduction.* Hillsdale, NJ, Lawrence Erlbaum, 1982.

15. Johnson MK, Zuck FN, Wingate K: The Motor Age Test: Measurement of motor handicaps in children with neuromuscular disorders such as cerebral palsy. *J Bone Joint Surg (Am)* 33: 698-707, 1951.

16. Beals RK: Spastic paraplegia and diplegia: An evaluation of non-surgical and surgical factors influencing the prognosis for ambulation. *J Bone Joint Surg (Am)* 48: 827-846, 1966.

17. Zausmer E: The evaluation of motor development in children. *JAPTA* 46: 247-250, 1964.

18. Zausmer E, Tower G: A quotient for the evaluation of motor development. *JAPTA* 44: 725-727, 1966.

19. Sutherland DH, Schottstaedt ER, Larsen LJ et al: Clinical and electromyographic study of seven spastic children with internal rotation gait. *J Bone Jt Surg* 51-A: 1070-1082, 1969.

20. Woltering H, Guth V, Abbink F: Electromyographic investigations of gait in cerebral palsied children. *Electromyography Clin Neurophsiol* 19: 519-533, 1979.

21. Berger W, Quintern J, Dietz V: Pathophysiology of gait in children with cerebral palsy. *Electroencephalogra Clin Neurophysiol* 53: 538-548, 1982.

22. Gottlieb GL, Myklebust BM, Penn RD, Agarwal GC: Reciprocal excitation of muscle antagonists by the primary afferent pathway. *Exp Brain Res* 46: 454-456, 1982.

23. Tardieu C, Huet de la Tour E, Bret MD et al: Muscle hypoextensibility in children with cerebral palsy. Parts I and II. *Arch Phys Med Rehab* 63: 97-107, 1982.

24. Ayres AJ: *Southern California Sensory Integration Tests Manual Revised.* Los Angeles, Western Psychological Services, 1980.

25. Sackett DL, Haynes RB, Tugwell P: *Clinical Epidemiology—A Basic Science for Clinical Medicine.* Boston, MA, Little, Brown & Co., 1985.

26. Bergman AB, Stamm SJ: The morbidity of cardiac nondisease in schoolchildren. *N Eng J Med* 276: 1008-1013, 1967.

27. Krebs DE, Edelstein JE, Fishman S: Reliability of observational kinematic gait analysis. *Phys Ther* 65: 1027-1033, 1985.

28. Haley SM, Harris SR, Tada WL et al: Item reliability of the Movement Assessment of Infants. *Phys Occup Ther in Pediatr* 6: 21-39, 1986.

29. Harris SR, Smith LH, Krukowski L: Goniometric reliability for a child with spastic quadriplegia. *J Pediatr Orthoped* 5: 348-351, 1985.

30. Pendya S, Florence JM, King WM et at: Reliability of goniometric measurements in patients with Duchenne muscular dystrophy. *Phys Ther* 65: 1339-1342, 1985.

31. Lewko JH: Current practices in evaluating motor behavior of disabled children. *Am J Occup Ther* 30: 413-419, 1976.

32. Brazelton TB: *Neonatal Behavior Assessment Scale*, 2nd ed. Philadelphia, JB Lippincott Co., 1984.

KEY POINTS

1. Progress has been slow in developing standardized tests in occupational and physical therapy for several reasons including the tremendous complexity in sorting out the constructs that need to be measured.
2. Reasons for the lack of universally agreed upon tests in the therapies include the service orientation of the professions, isolation of academics from clinicians, and poor access to funding resources.
3. Therapists in the field report poor knowledge of tests, inappropriate use of standardized tests, and heavy reliance on self-generated checklists.
4. The major advantages of standardized tests are their objectivity, quantitative scores, contribution to communication among professionals, and cost/benefit ratio in application to practice.
5. Because of the unreliability of clinical judgments, formal tests are needed to supplement diagnostic capabilities and provide objective measures of treatment efficacy.
6. Development of instruments is needed to assess motor performance, quality of movement, sensorimotor performance, occupational behavior, functional capacities, and developmental disabilities.
7. Current trends suggest that therapists are becoming increasingly interested in using standardized tests and in conducting research to develop new tests.
8. A combined effort by therapists and researchers in test development will lead to the advancement of a scientific body of knowledge, support for upgrading education and practice, increased financial resources for research, improved status of the professions, and increased communication with other fields.

Chapter 2

Planning the Initial Version

Bette R. Bonder

Problems are only opportunities in work clothes.

— *Henry J. Kaiser (1882-1967)*

INTRODUCTION

Careful planning is essential to successful test development. Helmstadter notes that this is the most important step, but one frequently overlooked.[1] The planning phase may seem time-consuming, but in the long run it is time well invested. Considerable thought must be given to each aspect of development. The process is a complex one but adequate attention to planning is vital to an acceptable outcome.

Planning involves determination of the test's purpose: reviewing the relevant literature; development of a table of specifications which leads to content selection; formulation of the initial constructs into test items; designing the normative, reliability, and validity studies; consideration of ethical issues; and funding the project. These steps are interrelated; the development process involves movement back and forth among these tasks as new information is obtained. Though discussed here in linear fashion, the process is an interactive one.

Bette R. Bonder, PhD, OTR, is a consultant to Cleveland Works, Inc., 468 Sandhurst Dr., Highland Heights, OH 44143.

FORMULATING THE IDEA

The Purpose of the Test

Most therapists in clinical practice are all too familiar with the need for standardized instruments. In the assessment of clients, they frequently resort to "homemade" measures with no assurance that these instruments measure what they need to know, or how performance compares across individuals. Even if clinical judgments confirm the findings, third party payers or clients and their family members may question outcomes. Thus, the impetus for instrument development is often a direct clinical concern, i.e., "If only there was a standardized instrument to measure . . ."

This perceived need by therapists for objective tools must be carefully delineated[2] into specific questions prior to initiating the development of a new test. The test development process is most effective when theory is based, that is, centered on an identifiable philosophy or model. Boundaries of the test must be identified prior to item development. The domains and constructs to be measured must be specified.[3] At this point, the purpose may be stated rather generally, e.g., "The instrument will measure Activities of Daily Living (ADL) as an indicator of role function." Because no single instrument can measure everything, the purpose must be limited in some manageable fashion. It is unrealistic to assume that an overall measure of "functional level" can be developed, but much more feasible to identify some component of function, e.g., activities of daily living, or strength of the upper extremity, as a focus for assessment.

Once the broad parameters of the instrument and the population have been identified, objectives for the measure can be stated.[3] These are general statements of purpose, e.g., "The test will measure ability to perform ADL activities among community-living elderly individuals." An instrument will probably have more than one objective, though all the objectives should be related to each other through the theoretical base of the test. The objectives form the framework for content identification.

Operational Definitions

The next step in planning is preliminary development of *operational definitions*. The purpose of the instrument should be stated in broad terms defining the domain or constructs to be measured using operational definitions.[3] Operational definitions are clear statements of the observable parameters of each construct or function to be measured. In other words, the construct to be measured must be described in terms of observable and quantifiable behaviors. It is helpful to avoid obscure or unduly complicated definitions which may be difficult for users to interpret, thereby posing a potential threat to the test's reliability and validity.

For some constructs the definition process is relatively simple. For example, performance of activities of daily living (ADL) can be observed. Other constructs may be less overt, however. Sensory integration is an internal process which cannot be directly witnessed. It can only be inferred from behaviors which are thought to be associated with it. Operational definitions of sensory integration address the skills assumed to reflect its presence or absence.

Definition of terms ordinarily begins with review of pertinent literature, particularly theoretical and research papers which discuss the construct of interest. If, for instance, one is interested in the sensory-integrative syndrome of tactile defensiveness, the literature about etiology and behavioral manifestations of tactile defensiveness must be examined. Papers which discuss observable, quantifiable behaviors are especially useful. If for instance tactile defensiveness is demonstrated by rapid withdrawal from sudden touch, this would then be incorporated into the operational definition. The *Miller Assessment for Preschoolers* (MAP)[4] provides an operational definition for "preacademic problems" which distinguishes it from learning disabilities or from school problems. The definition is the result of a careful synthesis of related literature.

Operational definitions are most successfully formulated when behaviors are viewed from several points of view. The statement "displays adequate pincer grasp" is an example of a poorly (nonoperationally) defined trait. Therapists or testers should choose different behaviors that might qualify as "adequate pincer grasp," such as picking up a raisin, moving a peg in a pegboard, or buttoning a shirt. In this case, three therapists might disagree that the child "passed" the item "adequate pincer grasp," depending upon which of the three behaviors they selected for observation. If consensus by experts can be reached on what behaviors qualify as "adequate pincer grasp" then an increase in the rate of agreement in observations would probably be manifested.

Disagreements between professionals often reflect differences in operational definitions of the behaviors in question. Consider, for example, a physical educator and a therapist who are observing a child engaged in crab walking. The physical educator is likely to comment on the good balance and coordination exhibited by the student. The therapist might simultaneously be considering the proprioceptive nature of the position and the joint integrity required to maintain the position over time. The scoring criteria must be operationally defined based upon the intended test users.

Many behaviors can be clearly defined and measured, but *purposeful behavior* is usually more complex and therefore difficult to separate into component parts for evaluation. The organization of purposeful activity into components of performance can contribute to the operational definition. For example, consider the errors that might occur if a test of toothbrushing competence only measured tube squeezing, lid removal, grip, and ability to repeat the brush movement, without ever observing the person's ability to do the entire task in its proper context. Yet, it is a difficult task to operationally define adequate toothbrushing so that all observers would reach the same conclusions. These considerations must be carefully examined by the test developer who aspires to measure "toothbrushing."

Carefully operationalizing definitions for all items will have a significant impact on both the reliability and validity of items (see Chapters 6 and 7).

After the items have been compiled, they must be carefully reviewed to ensure that objective scoring is possible. This requires operationalizing all definitions needed for obtaining scores. "Pass" versus "fail" criteria must be carefully noted. For example, when considering the number of seconds a child can stand on one foot, the operational definition of what a child needs to do to "pass" the item, might include posture of the trunk, position(s) of the raised leg, prior positioning of the arms, and position of the foot on the floor. Without clear specifications, different examiners might score the item differently, having varying expectations for passing criteria. This difference would also have a considerable impact on test reliability (see Chapter 6).

Population Intended

Once the construct is operationally defined, the population for which the instrument is intended must be specified.[3] This procedure involves identifying which group, and what portion of the group is to be measured.[5] It is a necessary step in determining the scope of items, prior to later standardization. Items which are appropriate for adolescents may be quite different from those for young children, and an attempt to serve both populations may lead to an instrument which serves neither. Given the complexities of test development, a conservative approach is wise in delineating the boundaries of the population.

REVIEWING THE LITERATURE

Review of the literature serves a number of important functions. First, if an instrument already exists for the desired purpose, it will be discovered,[3] eliminating the need to develop the proposed new measure. A good starting point for this portion of the review is *Buros Mental Measurements Yearbook*.[6] This reference book provides a compendium of reviews of published instruments, and details information about availability, content, administration, reliability, and validity. For most of the tests, several reviews by experts in tests and measurements are included as well as bibliographies of additional studies completed with the instruments. There are now a number of similar guides to tests in print such as *Test Critiques*.[7] Many good instrument reviews are also found in professional journals such as *Physical & Occupational Therapy in Pediatrics, Exceptional Children,*[8] *News on Tests,*[9] *Journal of Psychoeducational Assessment,*[10] and *Psychometrika*.[11] Catalogs from test publishers also provide useful psychometric information (*Buros Mental Measurements Yearbook*[6] provides complete listings of test publishers, addresses, and phone numbers).

Another purpose for a literature search is the refining of operational definitions and further clarification of the test's purpose and scope. Locating related instruments may be helpful in narrowing the focus of the new instrument. Further, other tests may provide guidance about operational definitions, since definitions for the intended test may be similar to those in other instruments.

The third goal of a literature search is further clarification of a theoretical framework upon which continued development can be based. Instruments which are theory based are likely to provide more relevant, coherent information for a specified purpose than instruments reflecting conglomerations of loosely related items. The theory base provides a foundation for the next steps in development. Tests such as the *Sensory Integration and Praxis Test* (SIPT)[12] and the MAP[4] provide extensive discussions of theoretical frameworks. This information assists the user in understanding and interpreting the test's purpose and results. On the other hand, the *Bayley Scales of Infant Development*[13] does not provide such a discussion, and thus the test user has the total responsibility for interpretation of test results and inferences regarding what domain of behavior is implicated by particular scores.

The final goal of the literature review is to glean useful suggestions about methodology for item design, test development, and reliability and validity studies. Reading about procedures used with other assessments in their development process can provide considerable guidance, and allow the researcher to avoid mistakes made by others.

The literature review may alter the initial plan. It can be anticipated that as the search progresses, changes will occur in the scope of the instrument, operational definitions, and plans for further investigation. These modifications can vastly influence later stages of development.

IDENTIFICATION OF SPECIFIC CONTENT FOR ITEMS

Having completed these steps, it is now possible to begin to identify specific content. Wiggins[14] suggests that there are three possible approaches to content selection: *analytic, empirical,* and *rational.* The first, analytic, is a theory based approach which holds that items are chosen on the basis of their relationship to a theoretical construct. If sensory integration theory indicates that age related fine motor skills are important, then the test would include items which measure those skills on an age based scale.

Using the second approach, empirical, the researcher identifies an existing measure of a closely related construct, and selects items which appear to be associated with that measure. The items which correlate most significantly with the related construct would be retained. For example, if a test of work readiness was to be developed, evaluations of successful and unsuccessful workers might be reviewed, and items selected which appear related to the divergent groups. Items would then be administered to known effective and ineffective employees, and those retained which discriminate between the two groups.

The third method is the rational, or sequential system approach[15] which integrates the analytic and empirical approaches. Currently, this model is the most prevalent as it combines theory with observation.

THE TABLE OF SPECIFICATIONS

One common method for specifying test content and organizing specific objectives prior to selection of items is the development of a *table of specifications*.[16] The table of specifications is a matrix which provides information about each item on the assessment, and what corresponding domain of development is assessed. The table of specifications is a two-way table and is generally constructed in one of two formats.

In the first format, the matrix has domains to be measured in one direction with age groups in the other direction. This type of table of specifications provides a blueprint for the number of items needed at each age to measure each construct or trait. The test developer then assigns percentages to each cell which reflect the importance of measuring each domain at each age.

In the second format, one dimension represents the broad constructs or traits which the test is intended to measure and the other dimension denotes the skills or behaviors that are representative of those constructs or traits (generally in the form of test items). Freeman[5] identifies these axes as the gross variable, and the operational level. The test developer notes which skill or behavior is intended to measure each construct or trait. This second type of table of specifications is completed after items have been selected. it is recommended that, whenever possible, the table of specifications be developed by a panel of experts, and that each domain be rated according to its relative value in assessing various ages to be included on the test.[17]

Tables 1 and 2 demonstrate two variations of tables of specifications. Table 1 is the table of specifications from which the *Miller Infant and Toddler Screen* (now called the *Miller Infant and Toddler Test* or MITT)[18] motor subtest is currently being constructed. It demonstrates the relative importance of each domain of motor performance at each age as determined by a panel of experts. Table 2 is the table of specifications from the MAP[4] which delineates for each item the domain of development that the item is intended to measure.

ITEM FORMAT

Item Type

Item format must also be identified at this time. Many measures of interest to therapists use *performance items*. Performance items require the individual to perform a specific task in a particular fashion, and provide instructions to the tester about scoring either on observation of performance or some specified outcome. Psychomotor scales to score such observations in a standard fashion are discussed in more detail in Greenstein[19] and Harrow.[20]

Observational measures may also be effective items for measurement of physical performance. Observational items require the tester to watch the subject in a natural setting, and rate behaviors which occur in that setting. For performance items or observational items, scoring will be specified either on some numerical scale, or on the basis of a qualitative description or rating. For example, an activities of daily living assessment might require that a subject put on a specific garment (performance), or that the tester watch during the time the subject would normally dress (observational). In both

TABLE 1. Table of Specifications for the Motor Domain Subtest of the Miller Infant and Toddler Test (MITT)[18]

Percentage of Items in Each Subdomain in Each Age Group

Age Group	1	2	3	4	5	6	7	8	9
Age in Months	0-4	5-8	9-12	13-16	17-20	21-24	25-28	29-32	33-36
Neurological Foundations	50%	40%	25%	20%	15%	15%	10%	10%	10%
Stability	25	25	25	25	20	20	20	20	15
Mobility	20	25	30	30	35	30	30	30	30
Motor Organization	5	10	20	25	30	35	40	40	45

TABLE 2. Table of Specifications for the Miller Assessment for Preschoolers[1]

	Quantifiable Behaviors	Tower	Sequencing	Block Designs	Block Tapping	Stereognosis	Finger Local.	Object Memory	Puzzles	Figure-Ground	Draw-a-Person	Motor Accuracy	Vertical Writing	Hand-to-Nose	Romberg	Stepping	Walks Line	Supine Flexion	Kneel-Stand	Im. of Postures	Tongue Movements	Rap. Alt. Movements	Maze	General Information	Follow Directions	Articulation	Sentence Repetition	Digit Repetition	Beh. During Testing	Supp. Observations	Tryout Edition
Foundations	Sense of Position and Movement												X	X	X	X	X					X								X	
	Sense of Touch					X	X																							X	
	Components of Basic Movement Patterns																	X	X											X	
	Ocular Reactions																													X	X
	Body Scheme										X									X	X										
Coordination	Gross Motor																X			X		X									
	Fine Motor	X		X							X	X	X																		
	Oral Motor																				X					X					
	Articulation																									X					

Verbal Cognition

- Verbal Problem Solving
- Classification/Association
- Comprehension/Auditory Processing
- Following Directions
- Quantitative Concepts
- Prepositions/Spatial Relationships
- Oral Expressive Language (vocabulary, syntax, etc.)
- Sequencing/Memory

Non-Verbal Cognition

- Sequencing
- Association/Classification
- Visual-Spatial Manipulation
- Closure
- Problem Solving
- Memory
- Visualization

TABLE 2 (continued)

Quantifiable Behaviors	Tower	Sequencing	Block Designs	Block Tapping	Stereognosis	Finger Local.	Object Memory	Puzzles	Figure-Ground	Draw-a-Person	Motor Accuracy	Vertical Writing	Hand-to-Nose	Romberg	Stepping	Walks Line	Supine Flexion	Kneel-Stand	Im. of Postures	Tongue Movements	Rap. Alt. Movements	Maze	General Information	Follow Directions	Articulation	Sentence Repetition	Digit Repetition	Beh. During Testing	Supp. Observations	Tryout Edition
Activity Level																												X		
Concentration																												X		
Ability to Structure Tasks																												X		
Need for Reward																												X		
Reaction to Separation																												X		
Interaction with Examiner																												X		
Verbal Interaction																												X		
Reaction to Movement																												X		
Reaction to Touch																												X		

instances, scoring procedures would need to be objectively quantified.

Another method of grouping items divides them into categories of *forced choice* (e.g., multiple choice or true/false) or *open-ended* (as is used in projective testing or essays).[2] Forced choice items require the individual to select from predetermined alternatives. This is the traditional true/false or multiple choice format which tends to be relatively simple to score with easily quantified scores. Although highly objective, forced choice items limit the range of possible responses. Open-ended items may yield much more information, but are more difficult to quantify due to the greater range of possible responses.

Similarly, item scoring may be either *objective or subjective*. Objective items have a widely agreed upon correct answer. A client being evaluated either can or cannot put on a shirt. Similarly, there is a correct selection when one is asked to match a design as in the SIPT.[12] Sentence completion tasks, one form of open-ended testing, have more subjective scoring, and allow for more ambiguous, creative, or idiosyncratic responses.

Each of these item formats has advantages and disadvantages. Objective items, such as forced choice, have the benefit of correct and easily scored responses, but may yield less information than open-ended, more subjective items. Since open-ended items require a more subjective scoring system, they are generally less reliable. Paper and pencil items may provide more information about knowledge, while performance items may yield more information about skill. The test developer must give careful consideration to the purpose of the test and the outcomes desired before selecting an item format.

Item Response Format

An additional decision facing the test developer relates to *response format*. *Multiple choice* and *true/false responses* are well known. Another frequently used format is the *Likert scale*[21] in which the subject is asked to respond on a scale of 1-5, or 1-3. Examples include ranking a behavior from "observed all of the time" to "observed none of the time" or "most liked by child" to "least liked by child." The format provides a systematic method for item responses, regardless of content.

Though it is beyond the scope of this chapter to delineate the considerations for selection of item and response type, a portion of the literature review should be devoted to these issues. The researcher must decide whether simplicity of scoring or depth of response is more desirable, and how important it is to quantify responses. A wide body of research is available which describes item types in detail and can be useful in selecting item format, or suggesting new mechanisms for obtaining information.[22,23,24]

ITEM DEVELOPMENT

Once a table of specifications has been developed, and an item format selected, specific items can be developed. There are a number of methods for accomplishing this task. Frequently, items are developed on the basis of *face validity*, i.e., they seem logical given the information desired. Items may be selected from literature on the identified subject, just as a biology teacher chooses test questions from the biology text. Items may also be solicited from experts in the field.

Theory assists in defining item content, as noted earlier, and items may also be developed based on those found in measures of similar attributes or constructs. Thus, in developing a sensory integration assessment, careful review of the theory which describes sensory integrative function may suggest item content, as well as existing measures of sensation, neurological function, or motor performance.

One special technique for item development is called the *critical incident method*.[25] This method involves asking either experts in the field or individuals for whom the test is being developed to identify the characteristic(s) most indicative of success or failure at a particular task, or most correlated with possessing or not possessing a specific attribute. On the basis of pooled responses, patterns may emerge which will dictate item content.

In development of an instrument, many more items must be generated than will appear in the final product. It is not unusual to develop 100 items to yield 10 useful ones. This process is necessary to allow for adequate piloting. Some of the items may be too difficult to administer or score, or fail to meet other psychometric criteria. It may be helpful to develop items in several formats and levels of difficulty in order to determine, through pilot testing, which items yield the most useful information.

At each step of item development, the involvement of a *review panel of experts* is essential. These individuals should be identified on the basis of their comprehensive knowledge of the area to be measured and of test development. The panel should assist in the generation of items and examine individual items to determine their potential value. An expert review panel can also be useful in an advisory capacity as the standardization process progresses.

When collaborating with an expert review panel, it is important to be as specific and structured as possible to facilitate their contributions. For example, it would be helpful to provide the panel with a descriptive rating system of aspects for each item (i.e., 1 = directions awkwardly worded, to, 5 = directions clear, will be easily understood by targeted users). This method also provides the test developer with quantitative information upon which to base decisions. An example of a quantitative form which was sent to subject matter experts to review items for the MITT[18] is presented in Table 3.

Prior to deciding which items will be retained or discarded, pilot tests must be conducted, and items analyzed for their ability to measure the desired attribute or behavior, and to discriminate between specified groups. (This process is further delineated in Chapter 3.)

Considerations in Item Selection and Administrative Procedures

Test items are determined principally by the purpose of the test and the target population for which it is intended. For example, if the aim is to develop a preschool screening test and the target population is preschool children, the complexity of the test-tasks would be designed specifically for that target group. In addition, directions for test administration would be worded appropriately for the target group.

The expertise of intended test users must also be considered in planning specifications for an instrument. A test instrument de-

TABLE 3. Example of Expert Reviewers' Evaluation of Miller Infant and Toddler Test (MITT)[18] Motor Items

	A	B
	Clear Picture	Good written description

Please rate each item (Columns A-E)
from 0 = does not describe item
to = 5 accurately describes item

SUPINE

1. Basic flexed posture

2. Head moving side to side

3. Head to midline hands together in midline

4. Hands to knees, head in midline

5. Hands holding toy

6. Head off surface (Anti-gravity neck flexion)

7. Trunk flexion with hands to feet

8. Trunk flexion with feet to mouth

C	D	E	F
Important aspect of development measured	Item will discriminate well between normal and problem children	Item is <u>not</u> culturally or sexually biased	Which domain of movement best describes this item 1 = Foundations 2 = Stability 3 = Mobility 4 = Motor Organization

signed for beginning therapists would consist of a different set of procedures from one whose primary users would be experienced therapists. Instructions and materials must be appropriate to the user so that terminology and techniques are compatible with users' background and expertise. For example, the *Southern California Sensory Integration Tests* (SCSIT)[26] was designed for therapists with advanced neuroscience knowledge, and a background in measurement and statistics. Test items and instructions for this test were designed with these premises in mind. *Developmental Programming for Infants and Young Children*,[27] on the other hand, was designed as a very basic criterion-referenced developmental checklist. Choice of items, administration instructions, and scoring procedures are suitable for entry level therapists.

PLANNING THE STANDARDIZATION PROCESS

The standardization of a test involves many steps. A large item pool must be generated and the various editions of the instrument pilot tested. Pilot testing is necessary to assure that instructions are clear, that items are effective, and that the instrument achieves the desired purpose. Validation and determination of reliability are ongoing processes. Numerous studies are necessary to establish that these vital characteristics exist to an acceptable degree.

It is essential to formulate general plans for the norming, reliability and validity studies during the planning of the initial version of the test. Although it is not practical to implement these on a large scale until the standardization phase, the studies must be *planned* as the initial version is constructed. The pilot testing and standardization processes are detailed in Chapters 3 and 4. Reliability and validity issues and processes are addressed in Chapters 6 and 7.

STATISTICAL CONSULTATION

The planning stages discussed require the input of a statistician, preferably one with expertise in tests and measurement or psychometrics. Advice on sample size and statistical procedures is invaluable, and will assure that methodology is appropriate. There are several mechanisms for identifying such an individual. Many health care facilities do research on a regular basis, and have research experts on staff. Local universities or colleges often have statisticians on faculty in the mathematics, psychology, or sociology departments who are willing to serve as consultants. Contact with a nearby occupational or physical therapy school may assist in identification of a consultant who is knowledgeable in the field.

ETHICAL CONSIDERATIONS

Research of any kind must protect the subjects, and instrument development is no exception. The research plan should specifically describe procedures which address: how cooperation will be obtained from sources on the subjects (i.e., school districts, rehabilitation centers, hospitals, etc.), how cooperation will be obtained from the subjects, and what precautions will be taken to ensure that the plan meets the ethical standards and legal requirements established for research.[22]

The test developer is ultimately responsible for all ethical practices in the conducting of research, including the treatment of participants by examiners, collaborators, employees, etc. Ethical practices involve respecting the individual's freedom to decline from participation; protecting participants from physical and mental discomfort, harm or damage that may occur from research procedures; informing participants of any potential risks; providing participants with information about the nature of the study; and maintaining the confidentiality of participants unless otherwise agreed upon in advance.[22] "The protection of individual privacy in . . . research involves two factors: the consent of the individual as to what will be disclosed to the researcher, and the confidential use of research data collected on individuals."[22,p110]

Test development research in pediatrics requires informed parental consent and cooperation. It is helpful if parents are spoken to directly about the project and provided with a written description. Specific information to be communicated includes: the time required of both the parent and child to participate in the project, the types of tasks the child will be asked to perform, the overall nature and goals of the project, qualifications of examiners, and how confidentiality will be maintained. Parental consent will also be required if photographs or videotapes are planned. Examples of a parent information letter and consent form used in the MITT study[18] are presented in Tables 4 and 5.

The test developer can avoid problems relating to confidentiality and possible invasion of privacy with careful planning of the project. Typical methods of gathering of data to protect confidentiality include: (1) collecting data so that no one, including the test developer can link the data to a specific child, or (2) using a system such as substituting numbers for names, so that no one can identify data for a specific child except for a person who has access to a closely guarded key.[22]

The *National Research Act of 1974* provides for the review of behavioral and educational research that involves human subjects by an Institutional Review Board (IRB). An IRB provides a mechanism for reviewing research proposals for the protection of human participants. Specifically the IRB examines potential risks as a consequence of participating in the research and determines whether the risks outweigh the importance of the information to be collected. In addition the IRB obtains assurances that the rights and welfare of participants will be adequately protected, that informed consent will be secured, and that the research will be reviewed at timely intervals.[22]

Planning for the protection of human subjects is also an important consideration when it comes to the search for funding. Many agencies require that detailed plans be elaborated. For instance, the U.S. Department of Health and Human Services requires that research proposals be approved by an IRB in order to receive funds. Exemptions from IRB scrutiny include: research involving normal educational practices which is conducted in established or commonly accepted educational settings, *research involving the use of educational tests if information is collected so that subjects cannot be identified directly*, research involving survey or review procedures, research involving the observation of public behavior, and research involving the collection or study of existing data.[22]

Projects exempt from IRB review by funding agencies are often still required to describe in detail the involvement of human subjects, plans for recruitment, potential risks, procedures for protect-

TABLE 4. Sample Parent Information Letter Used in the MITT[ih] Study

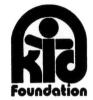

Foundation

Dear Parent:

Your child's program has been carefully chosen by the Foundation for Knowledge in Development to be part of a national project. The Foundation has received funding from the American Occupational Therapy Foundation to examine the developmental abilities of <u>normal</u> infants and toddlers at various ages. We will use this information to develop a test to help educators and health professionals detect problems in youngsters before they start school. Your child's program is supporting this project, and we hope that you will allow your child to participate.

We ask your permission to include your child as one of more than 200 children throughout the nation who will take this "test", a series of simple tasks and games. Testing time will be approximately 30 to 60 minutes. The testing will take place in your home or at your child's program at times convenient to your child and the staff. All testing will be done individually by a carefully trained occupational therapist.

Participation is completely voluntary.

Test Results

Because the test is still being developed, scores cannot be interpreted--we don't yet know whether a score is "low" or "high". Therefore, <u>no information about your child's scores will be given to you or to your child's program.</u> Results will be used only to develop this test and will be kept strictly confidential.

Selecting Children

Not every child whose parent gives consent will be tested. Instead, we will select children for testing so that they are similar to the U.S. population in terms of age, sex, race, community size, geographic region, family income, and parent's education.

The trained tester named below will be glad to answer any questions you may have about your child's participation.

If you grant permission to have your child tested, please complete the enclosed forms and return them to your child's program as soon as possible. Thank you for your cooperation.

Sincerely,   Name of Trained Tester:

_____

Lucy Jane Miller, Ph.D., OTR
Executive Director   Phone Number:_____

The Foundation for Knowledge in Development
8101 E. Prentice Avenue • Suite 518 • Englewood, Colorado 80111 • (303) 770-4818

TABLE 5. Sample Parental Consent Form

I give permission for my child to take part in the project with infants and toddlers being conducted by the Foundation for Knowledge in Development. I have read the Parent Letter describing the project. I understand that all test scores and information about my child will be kept strictly confidential.

_____
Child's Name

_____   _____
Signature of Parent or Legal Guardian   Date

_____   _____
Name of Parent or Guardian (please print)   Relationship to Child

_____
Street Address

_____   _____
City   State   Zip   Telephone (during day)

If you grant permission for us to test your child, please fill out the enclosed form which helps to provide biographical information about your child and your family. The information will be kept strictly confidential.

ing against risks, and why the risks are reasonable in relation to the anticipated benefits.

In the planning stage, it is advisable to utilize an existing IRB or establish a human subjects review committee which can be composed of, for example, colleagues, researchers, and representative parents and teachers. In this way, the test developer can ensure that appropriate procedures are incorporated into the design of the study for the adequate protection of the subjects when the study is implemented.

FUNDING THE PLAN

Clearly there are considerable costs involved in designing and developing standardized instruments. There is the time of the individual spearheading the project and the costs for consultants, copying, mailing, telephone, and staff time. Depending on the policy of the facility where the project is being implemented, indirect costs may also be a factor.

Consideration should be given early on to funding of the project. Frustration can be minimized if financial backing is obtained so that the project can proceed. This is, in itself, an immense project. If the facility or university has a grantsperson, advice should be sought during this phase of planning. In the absence of such assistance from a facility or university, other help should be solicited. This may be done, again, thorough a local university, particularly one which has an occupational or physical therapy program. Faculty there may be interested in serving as advisors or co-investigators, making available the resources of the university, including its grant-seeking resources.

There are a number of common sources of money, and some less frequently identified. The two most common resources are government bodies and private foundations. Local, state, and federal governments make grants to health care providers. Contact with government agencies concerned with the topic of interest (e.g., the local Agency on Aging, or the National Institutes of Mental Health) will yield information about current funding priorities, and, in some instances, about additional resources for funding. The *Federal Register*[28] publishes grant announcements, and some professional organizations regularly scan the publication to locate this information. While this is a daunting task for an individual, there are compiled summaries of the *Federal Register* that can be purchased on a subscription basis. *Federal Grants and Contracts Weekly*[29] is a good resource, as are The American Occupational Therapy Foundation (301-948-9626, Office of Professional Research Services) and the Foundation for Physical Therapy (703-684-2782).

Private foundations may be better resources for the novice. Local foundations often prefer to fund projects in their geographic region (e.g., the Retirement Research Foundation in Chicago or the Cleveland foundation). Other foundations grant money in particular areas of interest (e.g., the Robert Wood Johnson Foundation or Kellogg Foundation in health care and education). Universities may have grants available to their faculty and depending upon their individual priorities, school districts, hospitals, and state departments of health and education may fund pertinent projects. Occupational therapists are fortunate to have a professional organization (the American Occupational Therapy Foundation) which has a grant program which can provide sufficient funding to pilot projects. Local libraries, particularly college or university libraries, have reference journals and newsletters which list foundations, their funding cycles and priorities. (See, for example, *Foundation News*[30] or *The Grantsmanship Center News*.[31]) Foundations tend to have simpler application formats than governmental agencies, and many provide feedback to individuals who send letters of inquiry before full applications are developed. A personal touch in approaching foundations is recommended, as they are smaller and more accessible than governmental agencies.

Some corporations are also willing to fund studies. Insurance companies may be interested in the development of instruments which will assist in testing efficacy of treatment. Industries may be approached about tests which will be of value in determining work capacities. These funding sources are quite varied and require knowledge of the local business climate.

Successful fundraising is a skill which requires years to develop proficiently. The novice grant writer is encouraged to approach as many private and public agencies as possible in person. In this way interviews can be held with personnel to ascertain the appropriateness of that source of funding and accumulate valuable tips often excluded from application forms. Persistency most often yields the greatest returns.

SUMMARY AND RECOMMENDATIONS

Developing a norm-referenced test requires patience and planning. The planning of the project is complex, time consuming, and expensive with the success dependent upon the integration of careful attention to design, quality of consultation, and the search for possible sources of funding. However, a comprehensive strategy in the initial stages is the best assurance of the quality of the final product.

Adequate attention to planning requires that each of the steps in the test development process be carefully detailed at the *beginning* of the project. Many instruments are effectively developed to the point where they are ready to be standardized, but the test developer does not proceed. These instruments are extremely limited, as no inferences can be drawn from test scores generalizing the results. The considerable effort expended to develop these tools would be maximized if the therapists involved pursued the next steps.

The importance of test development to physical and occupational therapy, cannot be underestimated and is more fully described in Chapter 1. Survival of the allied health professions may rest upon their ability to document effectiveness, and such documentation cannot occur in the absence of norm-referenced measures with demonstrated reliability and validity. Numerous therapists have initiated the process of test development clinically by designing checklists or interview schedules. This is a good starting point, and *it is important to start somewhere*. Each small step has the potential to yield great benefits for the health professions and individual clients.

REFERENCES

1. Helmstadter GC: *Principles of Psychological Measurement*. Englewood Cliffs, NJ, Prentice-Hall. 1964.

2. Golden CJ, Sawicki RF, Franzen MD: Test construction, in Goldstein G, Hersen M (eds): *Handbook of Psychological Assessment*. New York, Pergamon Press, 1984.

3. Benson J, Clark F: A guide for instrument development and validation. *Am J Occ Ther* 36:789-800, 1982.

4. Miller LJ: *Miller Assessment for Preschoolers*. San Antonio, TX, Psychological Corporation, 1988, 1982.

5. Freeman FS: *Theory and Practice of Psychological Testing*, ed 3. New York, Holt Rinehart & Winston, 1962.

6. Mitchell JV: *Mental Measurements Yearbook*, ed 9. Lincoln, NE, University of Nebraska Press, 1985.

7. *Test Critiques* vol 1-4. Kansas City, MO, Test Corporation of America.

8. *Exceptional children*. Reston, VA, Council for Exceptional Children.

9. *News on Tests*. Princeton, NJ, Educational Testing Service.

10. *Journal of Psychoeducational Assessment*. New York, Grune & Stratton.

11. *Psychometrika*. Williamsburg, VA, Psychometric Society.

12. Ayres AJ: *Sensory Integration and Praxis Test*. Los Angeles, Western Psychological Services, in press.

13. Bayley N: *Bayley Scales of Infant Development*. New York, Psychological Corporation, 1969.

14. Wiggins JS: *Personality and Prediction: Principles of Personality Assessment*. Reading, MA, Addison-Wesley, 1973.

15. Jackson DN: A sequential system for personality scale development, in Spielberger CD (ed): *Current Topics in Clinical and Community Psychology*. New York, Academic Press, 1970.

16. Hopkins CD, Antes RL: *Classroom Measurement and Evaluation*. Itasca, IL, FE Peacock, 1978.

17. Ahmann JS, Glock MD: *Evaluating Student Progress: Principles of Tests and Measurements*, ed 6, Boston, Allyn & Bacon Inc., 1981.

18. Miller LJ: *Miller Infant and Toddler Test*. Englewood, CO, Foundation for Knowledge in Development, 1988, in prep.

19. Greenstein L: Psychomotor objectives in occupational therapy education. *AM J Occup Ther* 30:351-357, 1976.

20. Harrow A: *A Taxonomy of Psychomotor Domain*. New York. David McKay, 1972.

21. Likert R: A technique for the measurement of attitudes. *Arch Psychol* 140:52, 1932.

22. Borg WR, Gall MD: *Educational Research: An Introduction*, ed 4. New York, Longman, 1983.

23. Thorndike RL: *Applied Psychometrics*. Boston, Houghton Mifflin Co. 1982.

24. Hambleton RK, Swaminathan H: *Item Response Theory*. Boston, Kluwer Nijoff Publishing, 1985.

25. Flanagan J: The critical incident technique. *Psychol Bull* 51:327-358, 1954.

26. Ayres AJ: *Southern California Sensory Integration Tests*. Los Angeles, Western Psychological Services, 1980.

27. Rogers SJ, D'Eugenio DB, Moersch M: *Developmental Programming for Infants and Children*. Ann Arbor, MI, University of Michigan Press, 1977.

28. *Federal Register*. Washington, DC, United States Congress.

29. *Federal Grants and Contracts Weekly*. Alexandria, VA. Capitol Publications Inc.

30. *Foundation News*. Washington, DC, Council on Foundations Inc.

31. *The Grantsmanship Center News*. Los Angeles, Grantsmanship Center.

KEY POINTS

1. Development of test items must be preceded by identifying an underlying theoretical philosophy or model.
2. The purpose of the test should focus on manageable, quantifiable components of a function, rather than on general global abilities. Prior to initiating test development, the domains or constructs to be measured and the population for which the instrument is intended should be delineated.
3. Objectives form the framework for content identification. All objectives should be related to each other through the theoretical base of the test.
4. Clear operational definitions of observable, quantifiable behaviors which are intended to measure each construct or function must be provided. Obscure or unduly complicated definitions should be avoided.
5. The population that the test is intended for must be carefully defined. Success is more likely if a conservative approach is used (i.e., not measuring too broad an age range).
6. The literature must be reviewed to further define the purpose of the instrument, to determine if an instrument already exists for the desired purpose, to define terms and constructs, to clarify the test's theoretical framework, and to glean useful suggestions about item design and methodology for test development.
7. Specific content for items can be approached through use of analytic, empirical, and rational methods. The rational approach integrates the other two, combining theory with observation.
8. A table of specifications should be compiled to enumerate the number of items needed to measure the construct or traits in each age group evaluated by the assessment. Another form of the table of specifications is completed after the items have

been selected to determine which construct the item is intended to measure.

9. The formats for items include: performance versus observational, forced choice versus open-ended, and objective versus subjective scoring systems. Decisions about item formats must be made carefully before selection.

10. Types of item response formats for the test include: multiple choice, true/false, Likert scale, etc.

11. Item development and selection may be directed by theory, or based on items from other tests. The intended test users must be defined and expert consultation from representative users should be included in item development.

12. Many more items need to be developed than will ultimately be used to permit adequate pilot testing and discarding of items with poor psychometric characteristics.

13. The planning stages of test development require the input of a panel of experts and an experienced statistician.

14. It is advisable to utilize an Institutional Review Board or establish a human subjects review committee to ensure that appropriate procedures are incorporated into the design of the study for the adequate protection of the subjects when the study is implemented.

15. Possible sources of funding should be explored early in the planning stage. Information about funding opportunities can be gathered from professional organizations of occupational and physical therapy and local universities, businesses, and federal publications.

Chapter 3

Designing and Implementing Research on the Development Editions of the Test

Jan Gwyer

No one tests the depth of a river with both feet.

—Ashanti Proverb

INTRODUCTION

The development of a standardized test proceeds from the planning stage to designing and implementing pilot studies and the *Development Editions* of the test, tasks which are described in this chapter. The Development Edition of a standardized test is an important but often overlooked component of the test construction process. The Development Edition affords the test developer the opportunity to collect valuable information on test items and testing procedures. Eager to collect normative data on a test, the test developer might choose to proceed directly to large scale data collection and test standardization procedures, ignoring the opportunity to collect vital information through administration and analysis of a Development Edition. This chapter will highlight the contributions of

Jan Gwyer, PhD, PT, is Assistant Professor and Clinical Education Coordinator in the Graduate Program in Physical Therapy at Duke University Medical Center in Durham, NC 27710.
The author would like to acknowledge Susan Attermeier, MACT, PT, for her critical review of the manuscript.

43

pilot testing and a Development Edition to the overall development of a norm-referenced standardized test.

Pilot Studies Prior to the Development Edition

Numerous *pilot studies* lead up to the Development and Standardization Editions of a test. In general, they are smaller and more narrowly focused in scope than later research. Pilot studies are often termed, appropriately, the tryout phase. The tryout phase provides the test developer with a critical learning period for the refinement of ideas, items, and procedures generated from the planning stage. Depending upon the resources of the agency or individual, and complexity of the test, the amount of pilot testing necessary before a Development Edition can be constructed will vary.

The tryout or pilot phase allows for the flexible investigation of, for instance, the administration of a single item or a small group of related items to various children without concern for formal sample selection procedures. Various methods of administering and scoring items can be field tested. The general appropriateness of the items for the age group and population can be examined and materials field tested. Piece by piece, observation by observation, data can be accumulated and analyzed.

The overall goal of early pilot research is to field test as many items as possible. Then when the Development Edition is constructed, the test developer will have a preliminary basis for believing that the items will be psychometrically sound. The pilot process is less formal than the process used to construct and analyze the Development Editions, although it is conducted in a manner which has much in common with the description of constructing and analyzing the Development Edition later in this chapter, and the discussion of the standardization process in Chapter 4. Therefore, the information presented in Chapters 3 and 4 can be adapted to smaller scale pilot research. In designing this volume, it was determined that devoting a full chapter to the implementation of pilot testing would result in considerable redundancy. However, this is not meant to imply that pilot testing is not necessary or is optional. Careful design and implementation of pilot studies can lead to higher quality research at the Development Edition phase. In addition, pilot research can provide evidence to funding agencies of the merit of the work.

PURPOSE FOR CONDUCTING
A DEVELOPMENT EDITION

Once the pool of items for the test has been developed and the pilot testing of single items and groups of items has occurred, the next step in the process is implementing a study on the Development Edition. The Development Edition, sometimes referred to as the Research Edition, is similar to what the test developer believes the final test will be. However it is generally two to four times the length of the final test.

During the administration of the Development Edition, data will be collected from a sample including *both* examiners and test takers. This process ensures the selection of the best possible items and test administration procedures, for the standardization study.[1]

The data gathered is essential to modifying the test and is collected in each area delineated below. One or more Development Editions may be constructed and field tested depending on financial resources and outcomes of each study. If several Development Editions are administered the process would be similar each time.

Test Administration Procedures

During the Development Edition data are collected to evaluate the test administration procedures. The procedures outlined for administration of the test are followed exactly by the examiners. Using methods of observation, interview or questionnaire, the test developer gathers information from the examiners, and when possible, test takers, regarding recommendations for modifications in administration procedures.

Analysis of Item Characteristics

During this phase, a pool of items significantly larger than the total number desired for the final edition of the test are studied. Specific information regarding the utility of each item is collected and used to revise or delete items. This process provides specific psychometric information about items as well as more general information about item clarity, spelling, and grammar.

At times, particularly with young children, the length of the Development Edition can pose special problems. The test may have to be divided into parts and administered in more than one session. If this occurs, the research design should be counterbalanced for order of administration (i.e., the test developer ensures that each segment of the test is administered first in rotating order).

Evaluation of Preliminary Reliability and Validity

Finally, it is important in the Development Edition phase to initiate an evaluation of the reliability and validity of the test.[2] With the data from examiners and test takers, an initial analysis of the interrater and test-retest reliability can be performed. Evidence of content validity should also be gathered describing the relationship between the items and the domains of behavior the test purports to measure. Through careful sample selection, the test developer also gathers information clarifying the intended population for the test. Prior to describing procedures for analyzing data which is collected in the Development Edition phase, sample selection will be discussed.

SELECTING THE DEVELOPMENT EDITION SAMPLE

Sample selection procedures require careful consideration, as the information provided by analyzing of data from the Development Edition is used to select items for standardization. The information will be limited if the sample is biased. Walsh and Betz recommend that the Development Edition be administered to a "development sample" that are representative of the group for whom the test is intended.[3] A randomly selected, or stratified random sample will provide optimal estimates of how the items will perform when used with the intended population.[1] (Procedures for obtaining these types of samples are discussed in Chapter 5.) More common in research at the Development Edition phase is the use of a sample of convenience as described by Royeen in the development of a scale for measuring tactile defensiveness in children.[4] The more representative the sample in the Development Edition, the more confidence the test developer can place in the results obtained. Representative samples increase the likelihood that results will be similar to those that will be obtained on the larger and hopefully more representative sample during the standardization phase.

The size of the Development Edition sample is dependent on the specific purposes of the edition, but should be large enough to adequately represent special characteristics of the potential test takers. For example, if the test is targeted for both visually impaired and hearing impaired children, subsamples of both groups should be included in the Development Edition sample with numbers large enough to perform statistical analysis (n = at least 30, with larger numbers providing more stable results).

If the purpose of the test is to diagnose or categorize an individual by comparison of performance to a representative group,[5] then the Development Edition sample should contain test takers from the representative group. Most frequently tests are designed to compare an individual's performance to that of "normal." Therefore, the Development Edition sample should consist of a group of "normals" as well as one or more groups representing the intended test takers. The fact that the Development Edition sample is usually of inadequate size to produce normative data is not a concern. The data is only used for item selection and modification and is *never* used to provide norms.

Test developers should consider at this stage the possible effects of biased items. For example, to ensure that the test can be administered to minority groups, the test developer may want to oversample minority groups, providing greater numbers than would be required by Census Bureau statistics. By oversampling a large enough group of minority children, non-minority and minority performance can then be compared on each item. The test developer could then choose to delete items that were culturally or racially biased (depending on the goals of the test) at this point in the test development process.

TEST ADMINISTRATION PROCEDURES

Standardized tests may be defined simply as tests that use "standardization procedures for administering and scoring."[6] These standardized procedures allow the test developer to control the testing conditions to minimize the differential effects of factors that might influence test results such as: examiners, settings, time of day, and motivation of the subject. When such factors are controlled, the examiner can have more confidence that the results obtained are in fact comparable to the normative data reported for the test.

The Development Edition can be seen as an opportunity to evaluate the uniform testing and scoring procedures that have been developed. The test developer should design a Development Edition that makes optimum use of the available sources of information to evaluate test administration procedures. Examiners and test takers must both take (or use) the test, and provide the developer with feedback on the procedures.

Many of the tests used by occupational and physical therapists in their work with children are *individual tests* requiring a highly skilled examiner who concentrates on one child at a time. Another category of tests is the *group test*, which can be administered by the examiner to more than one child at a time. The tests may be *observational measures* of the performance (i.e., measuring a motor skill), or *paper and pencil measures* (i.e., performance of visual-perceptual skills). These characteristics will influence the type of testing procedures to be selected and the amount of uniformity that can reasonably be achieved.

The test developer should plan to use one or more strategies to collect information on the clarity of test administration procedures. Examiners may agree to be observed during the administration of the test. The extent to which the examiner followed the test administration procedures can be noted. This is the most desirable method of evaluating administration procedures, for in observation, the developer can observe the test procedures, rather than relying on what the examiner recalls doing. The developer's observations are not made with punitive intent toward the examiner, but rather to identify what instructions are not clear enough to allow reliable interpretation by various examiners.

If it is not feasible for the developer to observe all of the Development Edition examiners, a personal interview with each is essential. These interviews should cover any areas of confusion experienced by the examiner when using the test. In addition, a questionnaire should be used to gather the needed information on clarity of administration procedures. It should be completed by the Development Edition examiners immediately after administering the test to obtain the richest information. Tables 1 and 2 provide examples of part of a questionnaire that was completed by all examiners after administration of the *Miller Assessment for Preschoolers-Screen* (MAP-Screen) Development Edition.[7]

The following list identifies seven aspects of test administration

Table 1

Examples From Examiner Feedback Questionnaire

Used for the Pilot Edition Items on the MAP-Screen[7]

Item 1) SHAPE MATCHING

    a) Do you have any suggestions for clarifying/simplifying directions?

    b) Was the 45 second time limit reasonable?

    c) General Comments:

Item 2) FUNCTIONAL RELATIONSHIPS

    a) Any suggestions for clarifying simplifying directions?

    b) Were items generally ordered in terms of difficulty?

    c) Were any of the items particularly confusing?

    d) Was the discontinue rule reasonable?

    e) General comments:

Item 3) VISUAL CLOSURE

    a) Was the trial useful?

    b) Were items generally ordered in terms of difficulty?

    c) Are more specific time limits needed?

    d) Was the discontinue rule reasonable?

    e) General comments:

Table 2

Example of Examiner Ratings of MAP-Screen[7] Items

ITEM	Fun for Kids	Easy to Administer	Gives Good Clinical Info	Reliable to Admin	Reliable to Score	Recommend keep in test 0=no 5=yes
1. Shape Matching						
2. Functional Relations						
3. Visual Closure						
4. Object Memory						
5. Quantitative						
6. Problem Solving						
7. Sequencing						
8. Prepositions						
9. Sentence Repetition						
10. Digit Repetition						

Rate each item from 0 (does not describe this item) to 5 (strongly describes this item) in each category.

and scoring procedures that may be evaluated in the Development Edition. Test developers may identify aspects particular to their own test that also require close scrutiny.

1. *Statement of the test purpose and usefulness with client population*. This can be evaluated by direct questioning of the examiners or by observation of the test administration. Examiners must understand the purpose of the test and the client group for whom the test is intended. The test developer must provide a clear statement of the purpose and appropriate usage of the test. The Development Edition provides an opportunity to evaluate how well the test administration materials perform with the intended population.

2. *Overall clarity of administration instructions*. Score sheets should be evaluated to determine if examiners appeared to proceed directly through the testing procedures and understood scoring rules correctly. Incomplete score sheets may indicate points at which difficulty was experienced by examiners. If the score sheets appear correct, then more detailed information should be solicited regarding any ambiguities found by examiners in the instructions.

In particular, areas of the test requiring the examiner to proceed through a series of prompts or cues to elicit a behavior that was not forthcoming after the initial instruction or command should be noted. Test administration procedures must be as explicit as possible in these instances, using definitions or examples of what may be said or done by the examiner to elicit the response. If no additional prompts or cues are to be given, this must be clearly stated.[2] The more complex the allowable elaboration of instructions, the greater the risk of losing uniformity in use.

3. *Time limits allowed for the test*. If the test has a speed component, it is generally a good idea to have liberal time limits during the Development Edition.[1] This allows for collection of the maximum amount of information on the test items, since no items will be incomplete for lack of time. Examiners should be asked to record the actual amount of time required for completion of each item.

4. *The interaction of demographic characteristics and administration procedures*. The Development Edition should be planned to allow information to be collected from test takers and examiners of various races, ethnic groups, cultural groups, ages and genders. This is useful even if the test is targeted for a specific age or gender client group, since the examiners may vary on demographic charac-

teristics. In the Development Edition, the data should be examined to identify any instruction or procedure that will not be reliably interpreted because of racial, socioeconomic or gender factors.

5. *The use of testing materials.* If the test comes with all necessary materials, the clarity of the instructions for their use should be evaluated in the Development Edition. If the examiner must secure pieces of equipment for the test, this component warrants careful evaluation. Instructions should be clear enough to allow all examiners to select identical materials.

6. *Reporting and interpreting test results.* The administration procedures should clearly state how the results of the Development Edition can be reported to clients and parents without misinterpretation and with consideration for the rights of confidentiality. During the development phase, the method of reporting results should be established.

7. *Testing conditions.* A test developer must include environmental considerations necessary for development and use of the instrument. The use of tables or chairs or special equipment should be specified. The potential for auditory or visual distraction is a frequently considered factor. Also, space requirements for the administration of a test would be expected to influence whether the test can be used in a school, clinic, hospital, or in a private practice. All the factors should be carefully analyzed during the administration of the Development Edition.

If the test developer collects information on all or some of the above aspects of test administration procedures, the reliability of the final test will be increased. When conducting the Development Edition it is important for the test developer to analyze the perceptions of the test takers and examiners. This perspective will guide the test developer to make necessary modifications in test administration procedures.

ANALYSIS OF ITEM CHARACTERISTICS

Item analysis is performed by examining the responses on each item. The functions of the item analysis are to select the items that best fit the purpose of the test, and to identify items with poor psychometric characteristics.[8] The process of item analysis can be tedious, particularly if the test has many items and is administered to large numbers of subjects. It is unlikely that the task will be completed without the use of a computer.

Item analysis consists of examining four characteristics of each item: the *item discrimination* ability, the *item difficulty*, the *intercorrelations* between items, and the quality of the *item distractors*.[8] After scrutinizing the psychometric characteristics, the items will be classified into one of three categories: discard, retain, or retain with modifications. (Item difficulty and item discrimination procedures are further described in Chapter 4.)

Item Discrimination

In the theoretical framework of a test of cognitive ability, for example, intelligence or achievement tests, item discrimination is defined as the relationship between each item and the total score.[3] The ability of each item to discriminate between individuals who score high versus those who score low on the overall test is determined. To analyze item discrimination, the subjects are divided into two groups, high and low, based on overall test scores. Each item is then analyzed to determine if it was answered correctly by a large percentage of the high scorers. If this is the case, the item is considered to perform well in discriminating between the high and low scores.

The logic behind this analysis holds that persons who score high on the overall test and are said to strongly exhibit the characteristic being measured should also score high, or answer correctly, on any single item purported to measure the same characteristic. If there is not a direct relationship between scores on a specific item and the total score, then questions are raised with regard to whether the item is measuring the trait of interest.

The use of the total test score is customary as an internal criterion in determining *item discrimination*. However, the use of an *external criterion* may also be useful in determining item discrimination. An example of an external criterion is a diagnosis category or a score on another standardized test. In this respect, analysis of each item's discriminating ability would be completed by correlating the item performance with the performance on the external criterion.

For example, a test developer may be interested in creating a test that will be effective in identifying infants who will eventually be diagnosed as having cerebral palsy. Evaluation of the new test's predictive ability would involve an analysis of the total test score, any subtest scores, and the individual item scores with the external criterion, the diagnosis of cerebral palsy. The test's predictive ability will be improved by including only items which discriminate between the groups as defined by the external criterion.

The mode of scoring items influences their discriminating ability. Items that are scored with *nominal levels of measurement* (for example absent or present), are not likely to discriminate as well as items which use *ordinal* or more defined levels of measurement. Harris and Heriza[9] attribute the difference in the predictive ability of the *Movement Assessment of Infants* (MAI)[10] as compared with the Motor Scale on the *Bayley Scales of Infant Development* (BSID)[11] to this difference in the two tests' measurement systems. The BSID Motor Scale uses a nominal scoring system of pass/fail, while the MAI employs a four- or six-point ordinal scale. In addition to making the test more discriminating, the more discriminating measurement system on the MAI provides a more defined, qualitative description of the behavior of interest.

Item discrimination is calculated using one of the following three Pearson product-moment correlation coefficients: biserial, point biserial, or phi correlation coefficients. The calculation of these correlation coefficients is beyond the scope of this chapter, but is well addressed in the literature.[1,3,8]

Item Difficulty

An analysis of item difficulty notes the percentage of test takers who "pass" each item.[8] The procedure is useful to determine the level of difficulty of each item, and to identify poor items that may be too easy or too hard. Items can be eliminated that provide no information, for example those rated as absent or failed for all subjects. Decisions about selecting items on the basis of content are reserved until item difficulty data has been reviewed.

Intercorrelations Between Items

An attempt is made to clarify the relationships between items through a correlational study. This can be completed in two ways. First all the scores for items, subtests, and total test could be entered into a 2 × 2 matrix. Secondly, if the test is too large and this method seems cumbersome, items could be divided into sets logically by examiner, and only those items which the examiner hypothesizes are measuring a similar construct could be compared. The methodology selected depends on the quantity of data in the Development Edition.

This procedure can be used to eliminate redundant items and decrease the length of the test. It should be noted that when numerous correlations are performed, some correlations could be significant by chance. However, in general this technique is quite useful for eliminating redundancy.

Quality of Item Distractors

An analysis of item distractors is necessary for items that have one correct and at least one alternative incorrect response, found in multiple choice and pass/fail evaluations. When this type of item is included, it is useful to analyze the frequency with which each answer, the correct one and each distractor, is chosen by the Development Edition subjects. If no subjects or very few choose a distractor, it should be replaced with a more appropriate response. For example, a test administrator may present a child with four blocks, one red, one blue, and two yellow. The child is asked to select the blue block. An item analysis of the frequency of the correct response and of the distractors might indicate that the yellow blocks are rarely chosen. In this situation, neither of the yellow blocks is functioning as a reasonable distractor. Changing one yellow block to another color might improve the functioning of the distractors in this item.

The item analysis portion of the Development Edition gives the test developer some of the most objective information upon which to evaluate the proposed test. These analyses provide good estimates of how the items will perform with the intended group of test takers, and provide the researcher with confidence in using the test for its intended purpose.

EVALUATING RELIABILITY AND VALIDITY

Reliability

Many factors affect reliability, and the Development Edition phase can be used effectively to identify some of these factors, which, if controlled later through test administration procedures, will increase the reliability of the test. Kerlinger states, "Before they are anything else, measures of variables must be reliable."[12,p137] Therefore, the test developer should take advantage of the Development Edition phase to begin to evaluate the reliability of the items and total test being created. Many tests require the therapist to make observations of and measure variables or characteristics of clients. This process entails the interaction of a measuring instrument or test, and a rater or examiner. The reliability of both the items and test should be established. Two types of reliability should be evaluated during the Development Edition: *test-retest reliability* and *interrater reliability*.

Interrater reliability is defined as the amount of or degree of agreement between observers.[13] A test should be consistent so that two or more examiners using the test to assess the same behaviors will reach the same conclusions. Factors that affect interrater reliability include the clarity of the concepts being measured, the level of measurement used in the items, and the complexity of the testing procedures and scoring instructions.

Interrater reliability can be examined in the Development Edition phase by having examiner A administer and score a subject while examiner B observes and scores the same subject. The scores recorded by the two different examiners for one subject are analyzed to determine the rate of agreement between the raters. Further item reliability information can be obtained from examiner feedback regarding difficult items to rate or unclear directions for administering or scoring the test.

Test-retest reliability examines the extent to which individuals achieve a similar score when retaking the same test.[3] In the clinical setting, a special problem exists when subjects are unable to perform the same task in a similar way when retested. Factors such as motivation, motor learning, and the environment can cause variations in test scores taken at two different times.[14] An assessment of the potential stability of the items and the test can be made during the Development Edition phase by having the test administered to the same group of subjects on two different occasions.

Procedures for completing reliability studies are detailed in Chapter 6. The reliability results help the test developer decide which items to include on the final edition. Test developers sometimes make the mistake of waiting until the final standardization edition to complete reliability studies. At that point only post hoc information about test reliability will be available. It is prudent to provide as much reliability data as possible at this point in the test's development in order to ensure that only reliable items are included in the standardization edition.

Validity

Physical and occupational therapists use tests in clinical practice to measure certain characteristics of their clients, believing that this information will contribute to their ability to make decisions regarding the client. An assumption exists that decisions made using test information are more effective than decisions made without information.[5] The validity of a test "refers to the appropriateness, meaningfulness and usefulness of the specific inferences made from test scores."[2,p9] Therefore a valid test is one from which appropriate, meaningful and useful decisions can be made.

In the initial phase of test development, the test developer identifies the purposes of the test. Throughout the test development period information is collected that supports or refutes the use of the test for the stated purposes. The test developer should use the Development Edition period to gather information on test validity from the examiners. The type of validity most often examined in this phase is *content validity*.

Content validity describes how well the items in a test define the subject of interest.[6] Content validity is closely linked to the purpose of the test. If the purpose of the test is not clear, efforts to demonstrate content validity will fail because there will not be agreement on what content or domains of behavior the test should cover.[2]

Evidence to demonstrate the content validity of a test is usually gathered from individuals identified as having expert judgment in the subject area of the test. The initial evidence of content validity is provided by a detailed description in the table of specifications (see Chapter 2). The inclusion of expert judges to further develop the test plan, to weight the items, and to categorize the items according to the table of specifications provides the mechanism both to develop the test, and to describe its content validity.

It is customary to use a different set of expert judges than the group that developed the test, to review the table of specifications and evaluate the test. For example, the second set of expert judges might be the examiners in the Development Edition phase. Before using the test, the examiners might be asked to review the table of specifications, or to categorize some items according to the table. The test developer is interested in the degree to which the items selected represent the domains of behavior that the test purports to measure.[15] A test that demonstrates content validity, will permit generalizations to a broader range of behaviors.[3]

Collecting content validity information is an imprecise and ongoing activity. Demonstrating the content validity of a test does not require the computation of great quantities of statistics, but rather demands a systematic process of evaluation.[8] The test developer must also realize that evaluating the validity of a test is a continuing process. "Validity is not a static characteristic of a test,"[16,p2] and the evidence collected to demonstrate a test's validity describes the adequacy of a test for a specific purpose at a specific time. This type of information must be continually evaluated to determine if an existing test continues to provide appropriate, meaningful, and useful inferences. Validity is further detailed in Chapter 7.

The focus of validity research in the Development Edition phase is somewhat different than in the Standardization Edition phase. The individual items are usually analyzed specifically to determine their relative value. This information assists the test developer in deciding which items should be retained for the final version.

SUMMARY AND RECOMMENDATIONS

Having completed a Development Edition phase, the test developer will have compiled information to: evaluate all test administration and scoring procedures and make necessary revisions; evaluate each test item and retain the best ones; and begin to evaluate the reliability and validity of the test. It is possible that the developer would repeat the Development Edition phase with a revised test and a different sample of test takers and examiners. This decision should be made based on the test developer's confidence in the revised version of the test and funding availability. At some point the development period must end and acceptance of the test as the final version must occur. The test is then ready for a full-scale standardization and larger reliability and validity studies.

The Development Edition should not be viewed as an unnecessary step in the test development process by clinicians anxious to develop clinically relevant assessment methods. Every test will benefit from some form of Development Edition period, and the more rigorous examination of the item characteristics and the testing procedures, the stronger the test will be psychometrically. As Drotar suggests, test developers in the clinic or in the classroom should include time to conduct solid research and psychometric studies needed to demonstrate the "robustness" of the instrument across a range of populations.[17]

REFERENCES

1. Henryssen S: Gathering, analyzing and using data on test items, in Thorndike RL (ed): *Educational Measurement*. Washington, American Council on Education, 1971, pp 130-159.

2. *Standards for Educational and Psychological Testing*. Washington, American Psychological Association Inc, 1985.

3. Walsh WB, Betz NE: *Tests and Assessment*. Englewood Cliffs, NJ, Prentice-Hall Inc, 1985.

4. Royeen CB: The development of a touch scale for measuring tactile defensiveness in children. *Am J Occup Ther* 40: 414-419, 1986.

5. Mongomery PC, Connolly BH: Norm-referenced and criterion-referenced tests: Use in pediatrics and application to task analysis of motor skill. *Phys Ther* 67:(12) 1873-1876, 1987.

6. Wigdor AK, Garner WR (eds): *Ability Testing: Uses, Consequences, and Controversies*. Washington, National Academy Press, 1982.

7. Miller LJ: *Miller Assessment for Preschoolers-Screen*, pilot ed. Englewood, CO, Foundation for Knowledge in Development, 1987.

8. Weiner EA, Stewart BJ: *Assessing Individuals: Psychological and Educational Tests and Measurements*. Boston, Little Brown & Company, 1984.

9. Harris SR, Heriza CB: Measuring infant movement: Clinical and technological assessment techniques. *Phys Ther* 67:(12) 1877-1880, 1987.

10. Chandler L, Andrews M, Swanson M: *Movement Assessment of Infants*. Rolling Bay, WA, Infant Movement Research, 1980.

11. Bayley N: *Bayley Scales of Infant Development*. New York, Psychological Corporation, 1969.

12. Kerlinger FN: *Behavioral Research: A Conceptual Approach*. New York, Holt Rinehart & Winston, 1979.

13. Currier DP: *Elements of Research in Physical Therapy, 2nd Edition*. Baltimore, Williams & Wilkins, 1984.

14. Krebs DE: Measurement Theory. *Phys Ther* 67:(12) 1834-1839, 1987.

15. Connolly BH: Tests and assessment, in Connolly BH, Montgomery PC (eds): *Therapeutic Exercise in Developmental Disabilities*. Chattanooga, TN, Chattanooga Corporation, 1987, pp 9-19.

16. Sax G: *Principles of Educational Measurement and Evaluation*. Belmont, CA, Wadsworth Publishing Co Inc, 1974.

17. Drotar D: Implications of recent advances in neonatal and infant behavioral assessment. *J Dev Behav Ped* 8:51-53, 1987.

KEY POINTS

1. Pilot research can lead to much higher quality research at the Development Edition phase and can be used to convince funding agencies of the merit of the work.

2. The purpose of the Development Edition is to provide data for selection of the "best" procedures. It is specifically designed to provide information on administration procedures, item characteristics, and preliminary reliability and validity.

3. During the Development Edition, specific information regarding the performance of each item during test conditions is provided which is helpful in revising or deleting items. This process results in specific psychometric information about items as well as more general information about item clarity, spelling, and grammar.

4. A randomly selected or stratified random sample will provide

optimal estimates of how the items will perform when used with the intended population. The sample should include subjects from a group which represents intended test takers.

5. Test takers and examiners should be selected based upon their willingness to both take (or use) the test and provide the developer with feedback on the procedures.

6. More than one strategy to collect information on clarity of test administration procedures should be utilized. Observing examiners is most useful. Other methods of compiling information include a personal interview with examiners and a questionnaire completed by examiners immediately after administering the test.

7. The Development Edition phase allows for the clarification of: statement of the test purpose and usefulness with the client population, administration and scoring procedures, the use of testing materials, time limits allowed for the test, and testing conditions.

8. Item analysis should be performed to select items that best fit the purpose of the test and have good psychometric characteristics. Item analysis consists of examining: item discrimination, item difficulty, intercorrelations between items, and the quality of the item distractors. After reviewing psychometric characteristics, each item is either discarded, retained, or retained with modifications.

9. The Development Edition phase is appropriate for initial interrater and test-retest reliability studies. Factors which affect reliability can be identified and, if controlled later through test administration procedures, will increase test reliability.

10. To initially evaluate content validity, expert judges should be selected to review the table of specifications, evaluate the test items, and identify additional areas that should be assessed by the test.

Chapter 4

Standardizing an Assessment

James Gyurke
Aurelio Prifitera

What is well done is done soon enough.
— *Seigneur Du Bartas*
Divine Weekes and Workes (1578)

INTRODUCTION

The primary task for many therapists is to obtain answers to questions they have about a child's functioning. These questions are typically of the form: Does this child need services?; Does this child continue to need the level of services s/he has been getting? or; Has this child benefited from the services s/he has received? The most practical and efficient way to obtain an answer to any or all of these questions is to employ a standardized assessment instrument.

Standardized tests, as the name suggests, are methods that rely upon uniform administration and scoring procedures for obtaining a sample of behavior.[1] Implicit in this definition is that across each and every administration of a standardized assessment, the examiner attempts to keep testing conditions, item administration procedures, and scoring procedures consistent with guidelines set forth in the testing manual. The rationale for this is quite simple; by adher-

James Gyurke, PhD, is Project Director for Infancy and Early Childhood at The Psychological Corporation, 555 Academic Court, San Antonio, TX 78204-0952.

Aurelio Prifitera, PhD, is Senior Project Director in Neuropsychology at The Psychological Corporation.

ing to standardized procedures, the examiner is able to compare the results of one testing to those of another, and thus, provide meaning to those results.

Following is a discussion of the major steps involved in standardizing a test. This information is intended to alert the reader to the general issues involved in standardizing a norm-referenced assessment. Specific standardization procedures differ depending upon the type of test, the size of the standardization sample, and the amount of data being collected.

DEVELOPING THE TIMELINE AND BUDGET

Prior to beginning the standardization of an assessment instrument, a great deal of time and effort has already been spent in the pilot and tryout phases of the project (see Chapter 3). In fact, much of the work that goes into planning and implementing these initial phases can serve as a guide for the standardization phase. Efforts made during the Development Edition phase will have already determined which test items will be standardized.

The primary goal of the intitial phase of the standardization is to develop the timeline which will be used to guide the project. The timeline serves as the backbone for the entire standardization project and consists of three important components. The first is the target date for the completion of the project. When setting the target date, it is crucial to consider information pertaining to the size of the standardization sample, resources available, and the nature and complexity of necessary data analyses.

After setting the target date, the second integral part of the schedule is to establish dates for starting and completing critical phases of the project. Those phases include periods during which examiners are being recruited and trained, the sample is being recruited and tested, and the data analyses are being conducted. Weekly and monthly testing quotas, and realistic expectations of each examiner, should be built into the timeline. This will determine the number of examiners to be recruited and allows the test developer to monitor how sample recruitment and testing goals are being met on a regular basis.

Establishment of firm starting and finishing dates for each of these phases is critical because attention to such intermediary steps provides for realistic evaluation of resources required to meet the target date. The best way to ensure adequate support for the project is to plan ahead for the resources needed to meet the press of a critical phase and for how those resources will be secured. Without this support, it will be virtually impossible to complete the standardization in a timely fashion.

The third component of the timeline is communication mechanisms, a term which refers to mass mailings, meetings with consultants, meetings of staff, and any other activities which enable the test developer to make informed decisions about resource allocation and necessary adjustments to the project schedule. By building into the timeline an explicit period during which these communications are to occur, the test developer can aid the flow of information and avoid unnecessary and costly delays. A sample standardization timeline is illustrated in Table 1.

Although not part of the project timeline, an equally important aspect of structuring the standardization is the development of a budget, which in turn must be developed with full attention to the established timeline. General budgetary considerations should include: (1) the number of personnel required to standardize the test and the length of their service, (2) the materials that will have to be produced, (3) administrative time, (4) secretarial support, (5) computer/data processing resources required, and (6) any fees paid to subjects for participation. Of course, these general considerations will involve many specific details within each area, and many unknowns are intrinsic to the process. Because of the difficulty in estimating all the costs involved in a standardization, the goal in preparing the budget should be to estimate as accurately as possible the major costs. Once these costs have been determined, it is wise to take a fixed percentage, usually between ten and twenty percent, of the estimated cost and add it to the projected total. This "fudge factor" will safeguard against unanticipated cost overruns which may occur in any major standardization effort. An example of a budgetary form is provided in Table 2. Costs vary significantly depending on the scope and size of the project.

TABLE 1. Sample Project Time Line

<u>KEY</u>

P = Principal Investigator	ST = Statistician
R = Research Assistant	M = Measurement Consultant
S = Secretary	C = Subject Matter Consultants
T = Testers	

This chart designates the month that that activities will be accomplished and staff involved.

	MONTH											
ACTIVITY	1	2	3	4	5	6	7	8	9	10	11	12
Subject Matter Panel Review	C,P											
Develop/Revise Administration/ Scoring Procedures	P,R,ST,M████████████											
Staff Selection	P,R	P,R										
Staff Training			T,P,R,S									

Locate testing
sites, secure permission — T,R

Sample Selection, test sample,
reliability and validity studies — T

Staff Supervision — P,R

Data entry — S

Data Analysis — P,ST,M

Evaluation of testing
procedures and items — T,P,R   P,ST,M

Preliminary dissemination — P,R

Overall Project
Supervision — P

TABLE 2. Sample Budget*

PERSONNEL	**$ 63,525**

Fringe Benefits calculated upon 21% of gross salary and includes taxes, medical insurance, etc. FTE =full time equivalency.

Principal Investigator 36,300
    Annual Base Salary: $30,000   FTE 1.00
    Project Salary: 30,000   Fringe: $6,300
Research Assistant 18,150
    Annual Base Salary: $20,000   FTE .75
    Project Salary: 15,000   Fringe: $3,150
Secretary 9,075
    Annual Base Salary: $15,000   FTE .50
    Project Salary: 7,500   Fringe: $1,575

CONSULTANT COSTS	**$ 7,000**

Tests/Measurement Specialist (20 hrs x $50/hr) 1,000
Statistician (40 hrs x $50/hr) 2,000
Subject Matter Experts 4,000
    (8 consultants x 10 hrs x $50/hr)

CONTRACTUAL COSTS	**$ 41,000**

Project Testers (1000 testings x $40/testing) 40,000
    700 normal children, 150 at risk, 50 test-retest,
    50 inter-tester, 50 concurrent validity
Meals During Tester Training Workshop 500
Mileage in Driving to Testing Sites 1,000

OTHER	**$ 5,820**

Testing Prototype Materials 1,500
Promotion Costs to Locate Testers 500
General Office Supplies/Costs 1,000
Long Distance Phone 1,000
Mainframe Computer 2,000
Postage 500
    Mailings to parents, test sites, etc.
Videotapes of Test Administration 100
Printing 1,500
    Mailings, score sheets, examiner manuals
Concurrent Validity Tests 500

TOTAL CHARGES YEAR 1	**$ 138,515**

* Costs will vary significantly depending upon the scope of the project; qualifications of personnel, consultants, contract labor; geographic location; travel required; etc.

EXAMINER RECRUITMENT AND TRAINING

Successfully recruiting examiners to collect standardization data is a time-consuming, arduous task. Still, it must be emphasized that recruiting an adequate number of properly qualified examiners is critical for successful completion of the project.

The first and most critical criterion for selection of a standardization examiner is his or her qualifications, which includes appropriate academic coursework in assessment and other relevant content areas. This solid academic training is, of course, necessary for the examiner to fully comprehend the multiple issues surrounding individual assessment. Implicit here also is the examiner's thorough familiarity with the subject matter of the test to be standardized.

Equally critical in the selection of standardization examiners is the issue of the examiner's experience in administering standardized assessment instruments. All previous testing experience is a particularly valuable commodity because that experience has expressly provided an examiner with the opportunity to gain constructive insight into the more subtle nuances of assessment. This is especially true when the standardization sample includes children. Examiners who have ever assessed children will attest to the fact that, though the examiner's academic training was helpful, it was the hands-on experience of testing a child that most enhanced the examiner's skills.

Third, if the test to be standardized is undergoing restandardization or belongs to a class of tests which is presently being published, it is highly desirable to recruit examiners with previous experience with the particular instrument or class of instruments. This issue is simply a matter of economy; examiners who are familiar with the issues and objectives of the assessment being standardized require less training and monitoring than will a novice examiner.

Along with the qualifications of standardization examiners, the geographic location of the examiners must also be considered. For a national standardization, examiners must come from all geographic regions of the country, and represent both rural and urban areas. Adequate coverage within geographic regions facilitates recruiting, scheduling, and testing of the standardization sample.

Training of examiners also requires careful planning and execution. The primary purpose of training is to ensure *intertester reliability* in administration and scoring, provide a review of sample selection methods, and address the logistics of reliability and validity studies to be conducted during the standardization project.

Arrangements will need to be made for preparation of training materials (examiner manuals, test prototypes, scoring protocols, videotapes), space facilities, meals for testers during the training session, and the scheduling of "practice" children. It is helpful if a videotape of the test being administered correctly is made and shown during training. The videotape can also be used to teach scoring. For instance, after each item is administered, the tape can be stopped and testers can practice scoring each item as a group. Once adequately trained, intertester reliability can be established by testers viewing several subjects on videotape as the test is administered and then scoring the subjects.

Each tester should also be observed administering and scoring the test with practice children. A *"procedural" reliability* checklist can be developed to structure observations and feedback. An example of a procedural reliability checklist developed for the *Miller Assessment for Preschoolers*[2] is provided in Table 3.

Prior to tester training, sample prototypes of the test must be made. Because the test is to be standardized, it is essential that all materials be *exactly* the same. The materials selected at this point will continue to be used after standardization. Any significant change in materials after standardization has the potential to invalidate the normative results. Careful investigation at this stage will keep the costs of the final "product" reasonable and ensure that materials will continue to be available after the test is standardized. It may also be helpful to engage a professional artist in the preparation of the test prototype.

SELECTING A SAMPLE

Obtaining a sample for the standardization of an assessment instrument is typically the most time-consuming and labor-intensive phase of any standardization project. Before even one assessment is administered, a great deal of forethought and planning has occurred regarding all characteristics of the standardization sample.

TABLE 3. Example of Procedural Reliability Checklist for Selected Items on the Miller Assessment for Preschoolers[2]

TOWER **"THE BIG BUILDING GAME"**

_____ Blocks placed on table before child enters testing room.

_____ Demonstration model left standing until child begins building.

_____ Number stacked recorded correctly.

SEQUENCING **"THE PUT AWAY GAME"**

_____ Six blocks placed approximately 1" apart and 4" from table edge closest to child, parallel to table edge.

_____ Container centered behind blocks.

_____ Demonstration started on child's left side, all blocks returned to table for child to begin item.

_____ Suggested wording used.

_____ No clues given after child begins task.

_____ Pass/Fail recorded correctly.

BLOCK DESIGNS **"THE MAKE-A-BUILDING GAME"**

_____ Exact number of blocks placed in front of child.

_____ Model #1 taken down before building #2.

_____ Mirror image of design (from cue sheet) built for demonstration.

_____ Designs demonstrated quickly.

GENERAL POINTS:

_____ Card notebook set up for correct age group of child.

_____ Child's age determined correctly.

_____ Examiner adapts to pace of child yet keeps test administration moving along.

Accordingly, the first decision to be made involves the intended population for the test being standardized. A clear definition in terms of age, sex, race, and the like must be developed in order to assure appropriate sampling and norm development. For example, if the test being standardized is intended to be used for all children in the United States, between the ages of 6 and 16, it would be a waste of time, effort and money to test children outside the intended age range or geographic location. Once the population to be sampled has been defined, the next decision to be made involves the sampling procedure to be employed.

Because it is virtually impossible in most cases to standardize a test on the entire population for which it is intended, the only recourse is to standardize the test on a sample of the intended population. In standardizing a norm-referenced test, it is desirable to have the sample represent the population as closely as possible. Given this requirement there are two methods that can be used.

The first method is *random sampling* which refers to a situation where every potential sample of size N has an equal probability of being selected from the population.[3] Simply stated, random sampling implies that sampling is done in such a way that there is no bias in who is selected; every subject has an equal chance. Though desirable from the perspective that a true random sample is the best safeguard against introducing systematic bias into a sample, its applications are somewhat limited for large-scale standardizations. Because most populations have known characteristics (i.e., a certain percentage are female, a certain percentage are minorities, etc.) a limited random sampling from that population will likely yield a sample that does not accurately reflect the known characteristics of the population. In the event that population characteristics will not influence test performance, then the random sampling method is perfectly appropriate. However, if population characteristics are believed to impact on test performance, then the method of choice is *stratified sampling*.

Stratified sampling is a controlled selection for certain known characteristics of the population.[3] This method is the most commonly used when standardizing tests where the goal is to collect a national normative sample reflecting certain characteristics of the U.S. population which are thought to influence performance on the assessment being standardized. For example, a stratified sample will consist of a predetermined proportion of white males, between the ages of 10 and 12, who are middle class and reside in the eastern United States. After the stratification cells have been determined, the filling of each cell is done using a random process. An example of a stratification chart is presented in Table 4.

The initial step in securing a stratified random sample is to compose a list of all potential sources of the sample (i.e., for young children those sources might include day care centers, infant stimulation programs, preschools, church programs, YMCAs, rehabilitation centers, children's hospitals, etc.). Using a random numbers table or other appropriate randomization method, the sources should then be randomly selected. From a list of all appropriate subjects at the sources, individual children can then be selected randomly. Permission to test the children should be obtained at this point, in addition to demographic information on each child pertaining to the designated stratification variables (i.e., sex, ethnic group, community size, parent's educational level, etc.). An example of a biographic information form, to be completed by parents, is shown in Table 5. After reviewing these forms, testers can then determine which children should be tested to meet the quotas in each stratification cell. It is important to keep in mind that the more randomly the sources and the sample are selected, the greater the likelihood that resultant data will be error free and unbiased.

In terms of filling stratification cells, it is typically the case that certain cells, representing low incidence population characteristics, will be harder to fill than other, higher incidence, cells. Knowing this in advance, some preventive steps can be taken to ensure that those cells will not go unfilled. One step is to recruit these subjects through a professional search firm, such as an advertising company with a marketing wing or a large research organization. These organizations are skilled at identifying and locating these hard-to-find cases. Use of search firms tends to be expensive but time efficient.

A second alternative is to assign certain examiners, with access to a large subject pool, these cases to find. Chances are much greater that these examiners will be able to locate the difficult cases if the examiner is notified in advance that certain cases are a higher priority than are others. Though some cells will be harder to fill

TABLE 4. Example of Stratified Sampling Plan: Breakdown of % and N of Children to Be Tested in Each Cell by 1980 Census Information

		ETHNICITY				SEX		COMMUNITY SIZE			
REGION	N	White	Black	Indian/ Asian	Spanish Origin	F	M	Central City	Urban	Urban Fringe	Rural
Northeast	%	85	9	1	5	52	48	32	43	4	21
	420 n	357	38	4	21	218	202	134	181	17	88
North Central	%	89	8	1	2	51	49	28	35	7	30
	520 n	463	42	5	10	265	255	146	182	36	156
South	%	79	15	1	5	51	49	29	31	7	33
	680 n	537	102	7	34	347	333	197	211	48	224
West	%	78	5	5	1	51	49	33	45	6	16
	380 n	296	19	19	46	194	186	125	171	23	61
TOTAL	2000	1653	201	35	111	1024	976	602	745	124	388

TABLE 5. Sample Biographical Information Sheet for Completion by Parents

CHILD'S NAME	SEX	BIRTHDATE

1. CHILD'S RACE/ETHNICITY (please check one)

____ Indian/Asian   ____ Black
____ Spanish Origin   ____ White

2. FAMILY INCOME: (please check one)

____ less than $ 5,000   ____ $15,000 - $25,000
____ $5000 - $10,000   ____ $25,000 - $35,000
____ $10,000 - $15,000   ____ more than $35,000

3. MOTHER'S EDUCATION: FATHER'S EDUCATION:

____ less than 8 years   ____ less than 8 years
____ 8 years   ____ 8 years
____ 1 to 3 yrs high school   ____ 1 to 3 yrs high school
____ high school graduate   ____ high school graduate
____ 1 to 3 years of college   ____ 1 to 3 years college
____ college graduate   ____ college graduate

4. COMMUNITY SIZE: (Please check one)

____ more than 50,000   ____ 2,500 - 10,000
____ 10,000 - 49,999   ____ less than 2,500

75

TABLE 5 (continued)

5. Please write the letter corresponding to the appropriate group below.

_____ MOTHER'S OCCUPATION   _____ FATHER'S OCCUPATION

a) Managerial and professional specialty occupations: executives, administrators, engineers, scientists, health assessment and treatment occupations, teachers.

b) Technical, sales and administrative support occupations: sales representatives, cashiers, computer equipment operators, clerical, mail distribution.

c) Service occupations: police and firefighters, food services, cleaning.

d) Farming, forestry, and fishing occupations.

e) Precision production, craft, and repair occupations: mechanics and repairers, construction trades, precision production occupations.

f) Operators, fabricators, and laborers: machine operators, assemblers, inspectors, transportation occupations, motor vehicle operators, equipment cleaners, construction laborers.

g) Not in labor force: homemakers, students, seasonal workers, disabled, retired.

h) Unemployed

than will others, it is wise to attend to how all cells in the sampling plan are being filled so as to prevent an oversampling of a cell which results in a waste of resources. This can be accomplished by a weekly monitoring of sampling goals during which testers "report in" to the test developer of children tested that week. The test developer can check the children's demographic variables with the overall stratification plan to ensure the right number of subjects in each cell are tested, and to guide selection of additional subjects. Redirection, if necessary, can be given and testers can concentrate efforts in filling cells that have too few subjects.

A third method of sampling, one that is less desirable than the previous two, is obtaining a *sample by convenience*. As the name implies, this method is simply obtaining a sample in an expedient manner without regard to systematic sampling error. An example of obtaining a sample of convenience is a case where the assessment being standardized is a measure of depression. To obtain a standardization sample, the test is administered to the first five hundred patients seen at a family practice clinic. This sample, though providing data regarding performance on this measure, will tend to systematically overrepresent or underrepresent certain characteristics of the intended population.

Regardless of which sampling method is employed, it is vital to pay attention to the demographics of the standardization sample. Characteristics such as race, sex, socioeconomic status, age, and geographic location are factors which, if disproportionately represented in the standardization sample, will affect the normative data. For example, if a disproportionate number of females were included in the standardization sample of a test of preschool language skills, it would result in the norms being anchored at a higher level than if both males and females were assessed. A standardization sample should be reflective of the entire population for which the test is intended.

BIAS REVIEW

The final step, before data collection begins, is to review the items to be standardized for bias. A *bias review* is conducted to determine whether any of the items have *differential validity* for subgroups of the sample. The goal of constructing an item is that the item should discriminate among individuals based on the ability being assessed and not on some other characteristic (i.e., race, sex, etc.). Any item which does not meet this criterion is thought to be biased.

The process for conducting a bias review at this stage is straightforward. (A second type of bias review will be discussed in a later section regarding the analysis of standardization data.) At this stage, all items to be standardized are sent to a review panel which consists of several professionals with expertise in the content areas being assessed and the bias issues involved. These experts review each item from the standpoint of whether an item appears to be differentially valid for minority groups. Those items which are not felt to be differentially valid are included in the standardization with no modification. However, those items which are identified as differentially valid are reconsidered. When possible, the aspect or aspects of the item which were felt to be biased are modified or excluded and the item is included in the standardization. However, if the flaw is irreparable, the item is excluded from the standardization.

At this point, all preliminary steps in the standardization process have been completed. No further changes can be made in terms of the number of items or to the construction of the items themselves. The next step in the process is to collect the standardization data.

DATA COLLECTION

The *data collection* phase is in many ways the most critical and frustrating phase of the standardization process. The data are the raw material out of which the test is given meaning. This is also the phase over which the test developer/author has the least amount of control. It therefore behooves the test developer to organize and coordinate this phase as tightly as possible.

The degree of coordination depends upon the scope of the sampling plan. Obviously, a large number and wide geographical distribution of testing sites require much more logistic planning than few sites confined to a few locations. It is therefore important when deciding upon the sampling plan to consider how many and which sites are important for obtaining the information necessary for the test's intended purpose.

In order to make the data collection as manageable as possible, there should be an individual at each site who has administrative responsibility for the data collection. This can often be one of the examiners at a site. Centralized administrative control, especially with numerous sites, can become unwieldy and difficult to control. The coordinator might also be someone on site who has supervisory responsibility for the test administration and scoring.

It is necessary for examiners to have an identified expert to whom they can go for supervision on testing matters. In certain cases, it may also be a legal requirement that there be supervision of testing by a qualified or licensed professional in the state in which testing takes place. Such supervisors provide on-site quality control for test administration and scoring. Also, these supervisors can serve as trainers for the examiners. Having to train one person at a site who can then go on and train others is more efficient and cost-effective than the test developer having to train all examiners at all sites. If the number of examiners is relatively small, it may be preferable for the test developer to train all examiners directly.

The on-site trainer is one way of instituting quality control of testing and scoring. Such trainers can review testing protocols and assist the examiners in making needed adjustments in administration and scoring. However, it is also advisable to have some form of centralized review of protocols for quality control. A common practice is to have each examiner send in one or two practice protocols which are reviewed by the test developer. Further testing is not allowed until these practice protocols are reviewed and errors in administration and or scoring procedures are remedied. In addition to quality control, this has the added advantage of allowing the test developer to review many protocols and foresee potential problems which can be remedied. By continually monitoring test protocols, the test developer has a wider perspective on potential problems and can institute adjustments and modifications if needed.

Scoring rules are also best developed at a centralized location where a wider array and perspective of response nuances and scoring difficulties are available. By the standardization phase of the project, most of the scoring rules will have been worked out. Well-defined scoring rules are especially important for tests which have *discontinue rules*. An example of a test with a discontinue rule is the *Developmental Test of Visual-Motor Integration*.[4] "Testing may be discontinued after the child has failed on three consecutive forms. You may choose to continue, however, as it is often quite informative to see how a child approached the more difficult forms."[4,p38]

It is essential for proper data collection that examiners are well trained in scoring and the scoring rules are clear and well-defined when discontinue decisions are made by the examiners. The same would be true for tests which require the examiner to establish *basal* (starting) points for a test. For tests in which scoring need not be done by the examiner (i.e., where recording of response is sufficient), scoring rules are not an important issue for examiners. In this situation, the information which must be recorded to allow scoring must be clear to the examiners.

A necessary condition for good quality data collection is that manuals, record forms, and other pieces and parts be clearly written and easy to use and manipulate. Anastasi[5] lists these practical concerns as important criteria when evaluating tests. Such factors allow for a smooth administration, greater equivalence in administration across examiners, and allow the examiners to focus more of their attention to collecting the test data rather than trying to overcome the clumsiness of a poorly designed test kit. These considerations should have already been taken care of after the pilot phase, during the Development Edition, and during production of the standardization kit. However, some mistakes may occur or better procedures may become apparent after the kit has been produced. When this happens, the necessity and importance of instituting changes in procedures must be assessed and communicated to those involved in the data collection.

DATA ANALYSIS

The first step in data analysis is insuring that all data has been properly scored, the data files for computer analysis have been properly set up, variables properly labeled, and that the computer data files have been checked for data entry errors. Construction of a *codebook* is recommended prior to entering data which is essentially a "dictionary" of all data, terminology and abbreviations that represent the data to be entered into the computer for analysis. An example of a portion of a codebook is illustrated in Table 6.

It is also advisable to document all stages of data analysis since it is easy to lose track of what has been and what still needs to be done while one is in the midst of performing a multitude of analyses. The first step, typically, is to run basic statistics (e.g., frequencies, means, and standard deviations) on raw scores for variables of interest such as items, times and total scores. This also serves as an additional check to see if any variables have scores which are out of range.

Item Difficulty Values (p Values)

The index of *item difficulty*, or *p* value, is typically the first index calculated. This is simply the proportion of examinees who got a particular item correct. For example, if 75 out of 100 examinees correctly answered item 1 on a test, that item would have *p* value of .75. In general, items with moderate *p* values are preferable since such items provide maximal discrimination among examinees. However, many variables enter into deciding which *p* values one will accept and there is no one number or range of values that is best. Allen and Yen[6] present a detailed discussion of these issues.

For some items which are non-binary it is helpful to organize data into a *grouped frequency distribution*. To accomplish this, first the range of data is considered, then the intervals into which the data is grouped are selected, and finally the number of observations in each interval are summed. For example, if the item was stacking blocks and the range of scores was from 0 to 15, information about the number of blocks stacked at each age would have to be calculated before the proportion of examinees who got the item "right" could be determined. It is not until after all the data is aggregated that pass/fail criteria for non-binary items can be established.

TABLE 6. Sample Codebook

Page #	Card #	Column #	Item Abbreviation	Item Name	Description Minimum/Maximum	Example	Special Instructions
1	1	1-4	ID	ID#	200-340	A 200	First column is letter corresponding to region: A = Northeast B = North Central C = South D = West
1	1	5	TEST	Test Administration	1-3	1	1=1st, 2=2nd, 3=Intertester
1	1	6-11	DOE	Date of Evaluation	880100-880600	880511	Year/Month/Day
1	1	12-17	DOB	Date of Birth	820100-860600	830407	Year/Month/Day
3	2	25-26	LADR	Ladder	0-20	08	# lines drawn in 20 sec

				Reaction to Touch	1-2	1	1=Aversive Reaction 2=Normal
3	2	35	REACTCH	Reaction to Touch	1-2	1	1=Aversive Reaction 2=Normal
4	3	7	KICKBR	Kicks Ball R Foot	1-2	1	1=Fail 2=Pass
		8	KICKBL	Kicks Ball L Foot	1-2	2	
4	3	9-10	KICKBWLL	Kicks Wall	00-14	10	# kicks in 30 seconds
4	3	16-17	SUPFLEX	Supine Flexion	11-15	05	# seconds maintains position

Item-Discrimination Index

Such measures give an indication of how well items discriminate between high and low scorers on a test. For instance, an item passed by those who score low on a test and failed by those who score high on a test would be considered a bad item which should be discarded. A common method of calculating this index is by using a *point-biserial correlation* which correlates *dichotomously scored items* with the total score on a test which is a *continuous score*. There are other approaches and methods used for calculating item discrimination which again are discussed in greater detail by Allen and Yen.[6]

Factor Analysis of Items

Factor analysis of items is sometimes used as a method of determining whether items on a test are measuring the same underlying ability or trait. For example, if a test has two scales which measure motor and verbal abilities, a factor analysis of items should result in a two-factor solution. The verbal items should have high loadings on one factor and low loadings on another factor with the opposite being the case for the motor items. Factor analysis is described further in Chapter 7.

Bias Analysis

For some tests, certain types of biases (e.g., ethnic, sexual, cultural) may be suspected and of concern. The statistical treatment of bias is not the same as other types of *bias analyses* such as the type discussed above in the section on bias review. Statistical bias is also independent of the issue of test misuse or using a test which is not valid for a given purpose. The statistical definition of bias refers to "constant or systematic error rather than random, patternless error . . . the use of the term is quite distinct from its common 'lay usage.' "[7] Angoff[8] discusses several methods for assessing bias from a statistical perspective. In general, items found to be biased should be eliminated. Most of the biased items will have been identified and discarded at the Development Edition phase. Therefore, few items are likely to reveal bias at the standardization phase.

RELIABILITY AND VALIDITY

Establishing the *reliability* and *validity* of a test is a continuous process and impossible to thoroughly accomplish in a single study. Depending on the purpose and intended uses of a particular test, the test developer must determine which types of reliability and validity are most important to investigate during the standardization phase. The decision will also be influenced by what it is most practical to implement in consideration of the resources and time available, based on what information potential users will need to know to use the test effectively.

The reliability of a test refers to how consistently and precisely a test measures what it purports to measure. Two types of reliability are generally important to include during the standardization process: intertester and the test-retest. Test-retest data provides potential users with information about how much scores vary over repeated testings of an individual. Intertester reliability indicates whether consistent results can be expected regardless of who the examiner is. Particularly on tests which require subjective scoring or have complex scoring rules, intertester reliability information is an important issue to address. (See Chapter 6 and Anastasi[5] for a detailed discussion of reliability.)

Validity refers to how well a test measures what it purports to measure. Unlike reliability, validity does not refer to a single number. Test validation occurs through gathering evidence for a test's validity from various sources and through various methods. It is important to include validation studies as part of the standardization process to provide support for the test's intended uses. As many validation processes or studies as are feasible should be accomplished during the standardization phase of test development so that the results can be reported when the test manual is published. See Chapter 7 for a detailed discussion of validity.

NORMS DEVELOPMENT

Norm-referenced tests allow us to compare the score of a particular individual with a given *reference group*. The reference group is determined by the sampling plan of the standardization which has already been discussed. *Norms* allow for the determination of where an individual stands on the ability or trait being measured compared to those in the reference group.

In developing norms, several considerations need to be taken into account in order to determine how best to present the norms. For example, if developing a test of intellectual ability in children, the test developer would probably want to have age related norms so a child could be compared against same aged peers. If the ability being measured shows sex differences, the developer might want to have norms based on sex. For example, for height and weight, it is better to have separate norms for males and females than one set of norms for both sexes combined given the difference between males and females in height and weight. Other types of *subgroup norms* may be appropriate for given tests.

At times, *local norms* may be more appropriate and informative. For example, a school district may not be interested in how a child performs compared to a national sample of children on a given test but only compared to children within that school district. When devising the sampling plan it is important to have a clear understanding of what type of norms will be most informative for the user. One could have an exemplary sampling plan, excellent reliability, and yet have a test of dubious utility if the norms are developed in such a way that they do not provide the type of information that is useful to the user. (See Chapter 5 and Anastasi[5] or Cronbach[9] for a detailed discussion of norms.)

PUBLICATION

The time and difficulties associated with the manual-writing and publication phase of test development are often underestimated by the test developer. In this phase it is best to keep Murphy's Law in mind for if anything can go wrong, it will. In addition to writing the manual, record forms, scoring keys, pieces and parts (e.g., blocks, puzzles, etc.), and a carrying case for the final edition are produced. Other considerations include the attractiveness, ease of use, and quality of the materials which can require a considerable amount of design work. Further information regarding the examiner's manual is provided in Chapter 8.

SUMMARY AND RECOMMENDATIONS

The preceding discussion has highlighted the major phases involved in the standardization process and important considerations involved at each of these phases. Standardization endeavors, regardless of scope, require the orchestration of a large number of staff and subjects. The effort becomes a collective one composed of many "test developers" whose contributions range from entering the data into a computer to testing the sample to making final decisions about which items to retain.

One of the more important responsibilities of the test developer throughout the process is to establish ongoing, regular communication with project examiners, support staff, and consultants. This will ensure the timely completion of activities and reveal the need for corrective changes in project design. Mechanisms of ongoing monitoring and evaluation also provide an important aspect of quality control which will ultimately assure the value and integrity of the research.

The standardization process will differ from project to project; however, good planning and sound methodology will enable the test developer to complete this process in an efficient and effective manner.

REFERENCES

1. Mehrens W. Lehman I: *Using Standardized Tests in Education*, ed 4. New York, Longman Inc, 1987.

2. Miller LJ: *Miller Assessment for Preschoolers*. San Antonio, TX, Psychological Corporation, 1988, 1982.

3. Murphy K, Davidshofer C: *Psychological Testing: Principles and Applications*. Englewood Cliffs, NJ, Prentice-Hall, 1988.

4. Beery KE: *Revised Administration, Scoring, and Teaching Manual for the Developmental Test of Visual-Motor Integration*. Cleveland, Modern Curriculum Press, 1982.

5. Anastasi A: *Psychological Testing*, ed 6. New York, Collier Macmillan Publishers, 1988.

6. Allen MJ, Yen WM: *Introduction to Measurement Theory*. Monterey, CA, Brooks/Cole Publishing, 1979.

7. Reynolds CR, Brown RT: Bias in mental testing: An introduction to the issues, in Reynolds CR, Brown RT (eds): *Perspectives on Bias in Mental Testing* pp 1-39. New York, Plenum Press, 1984.

8. Angoff WH: Use of difficulty and discrimination indices for detecting item bias, in Berk RA (ed): *Handbook of Methods for Detecting Test Bias* pp 96-116. Baltimore, Johns Hopkins University Press, 1982.

9. Cronbach, LJ: *Essentials of Psychological Testering*, ed 3. New York, Harper & Row, 1970.

KEY POINTS

1. The first phase of the standardization process is to develop the timeline to guide the project. When setting the target date for completion of the project, it is important to consider size of the sample, resources available, and the complexity of necessary data analysis.

2. It may be helpful to build into the timeline weekly and monthly testing quotas for examiners and to establish firm starting and finishing dates for each phase of the project.

3. The budget should estimate as accurately as possible the major costs. It is wise to take a fixed percentage of the estimated cost and add it to the projected total to safeguard against unanticipated costs.

4. It is important to recruit an adequate number of examiners to successfully complete the project. The most critical criteria for selection are appropriate academic coursework in assessment and relevant content areas, experience in administering standardized assessment instruments, and geographical location.

5. In the training of examiners, videotapes can be used to increase consistency between examiners, and administration of the test with practice children can increase procedural reliability.

6. It is essential that all materials be *exactly* the same. Careful

investigation will keep the costs of the final "product" reasonable and ensure that materials will continue to be available after the test is standardized.

7. Sample selection initially involves clearly defining the intended population for the test in terms of age, sex, race, etc. It is desirable to have the sample represent the population as closely as possible.

8. A random sample is the best safeguard against introducing systematic bias into a sample, but its applications are limited for large-scale standardizations.

9. Most standardized tests use stratified sampling procedures. Whenever possible random selection should occur within each strata.

10. Preventative steps to identify and locate hard-to-find cases include the use of a professional search firm or research organization, or assigning the cases to certain examiners who have access to a large subject pool.

11. It is wise to attend to how cells in the sampling plan are being filled so as to prevent an oversampling of a cell which results in a waste of resources. This can be accomplished by weekly communication between testers and the test developer.

12. The least desirable sampling method is obtaining a sample by convenience. This method will tend to systematically overrepresent or underrepresent certain characteristics of the intended population.

13. Regardless of which sampling method is employed, it is vital to pay attention to demographics. Characteristics disproportionately represented will affect the normative data in the standardization sample.

14. The final step before data collection is to have experts review each item for possible bias to minority groups. When possible, the aspect or aspects of the item which were felt to be biased are modified or else the item is excluded.

15. An on-site trainer is one way of instituting quality control of testing and scoring. Such trainers can review testing protocols and assist the examiners in making needed adjustments in administration and scoring.

16. A common practice for quality control is to have each examiner send in one or two practice protocols which are reviewed by the test developer prior to further testing.

17. A necessary condition for good quality data collection is that manuals, record forms, and other pieces and parts be clearly written and easy to use and manipulate.

18. The first step in data analysis is insuring that all data has been properly scored, the data files for computer analysis have been properly set up, variables properly labeled, and that the computer data files have been checked for data entry errors. Construction of a codebook is recommended prior to entering data.

19. It is essential to document all stages of data analysis since it is easy to lose track of what has been and what still needs to be done.

20. Data analysis typically includes item difficulty, item discrimination, factor analysis, and bias analysis.

21. The test developer must determine which types of reliability and validity are most important to investigate during the standardization phase. The decisions will be influenced by the test purpose, practical considerations of resources and time available, and what essential information potential users will need to know to use the test effectively.

22. In devising the sampling plan, it is important to have a clear understanding of what type of norms will be most useful to the user.

Chapter 5

Norms and Scores

Sharon Cermak

There are three kinds of lies: lies, damned lies, and statistics.

—Disraeli

INTRODUCTION

Suppose that on the *Bayley Scales of Infant Development*,[1] Kendra, age 14 months, received a score of 97 on the Mental Scale and 44 on the Motor Scale. Does this mean that her mental abilities are in the average range? Does it mean that she is motorically retarded? Does it mean that her mental abilities are twice as good as her motor abilities?

The numbers reported are raw scores and reflect the number of items that Kendra passed. Since there are many more items on the Mental Scale than on the Motor Scale, it is expected that her raw score on this scale would be higher. These numbers are called raw scores and cannot be interpreted. It is not known what their relationship is to each other, or what they signify relative to the average child of comparable age. Raw scores can be interpreted only in terms of a clearly defined and uniform frame of reference. The frame of reference in interpreting a child's scores is based upon the scoring system which is used on the test.

Scores on psychological, educational, developmental, and per-

Sharon Cermak, EdD, OTR, is Associate Professor of Occupational Therapy at Sargent College of Allied Health Professions, Boston University,. University Road, Boston, MA 02215.

ceptual tests are generally interpreted by reference to *norms*. Norms represent the test performance of the standardization sample. They are established by determining what a representative group of persons do on a test. (This process is described in detail in Chapter 4.) In Kendra's example, her performance would be compared to the performance of the babies who were part of the normative sample when the *Bayley Scales of Infant Development*[1] was standardized. Thus, the raw score is converted to a derived standard score in order to: (1) indicate Kendra's standing relative to the normative sample, and (2) provide a way to compare Kendra's Mental Scale to her Motor Scale.

This chapter will address how and why various scoring systems for norm-referenced tests are established. Norm-referenced tests show how well a person does in comparison to an established set of performance scores. The statistical concepts related to the description of test performance will be addressed including measures of central tendency, variability, and types of distributions. Then a description of the various types of scoring systems applicable to standardized test development will be presented, including age equivalent scores, grade equivalent scores, percentiles, standard scores, deviation IQ scores, and stanines. Following this, the value and limitations of norm-referenced scoring systems will be discussed.

STATISTICAL CONCEPTS

Before proceeding to a discussion of the applied aspects of testing, it is helpful to examine some statistical concepts that underlie the development and use of norms.

Measures of Central Tendency

One way to describe a group of test performance scores is by examining *measures of central tendency*, that is using one number to represent the performance of the group. For example, to establish how long the average six-year-old can stand on one foot, 20 six-year-olds could be tested (see Table 1) and one number could be calculated to represent the average length of time.

There are three possible ways to describe this performance, the

TABLE 1. Scores of 20 Six-Year Olds on a Test of Standing Balance

Name	Score	Name	Score	Name	Score
Jolene	37	Daphne	19	Dae-Won	12
Anne	30	Megan	18	Joey	10
Randi	27	Ellen	17	Justin	9
Nicole	26	Nathan	15	Ani	7
Jose	24	Drew	15	Kara	6
Judith	23	Amanda	15	Marcia	1
Simon	19	Linda	14		

```
    Mean = 17.2    Sum of Scores ÷ Number of Children

    Mode = 15      Score which occurs most frequently

 Median = 16       The score which is ranked in the middle
```

mean, median, and *mode.* The *mean* is the arithmetic average which is computed by adding the scores of all the children and dividing it by the number of children tested, in this case, 20. In the example given in Table 1, the mean is 17.2 seconds.

The mean is the most common, and generally the most useful, measure of central tendency. However, a possible disadvantage of the mean is that if one score is extremely different from the others, this one score will distort or skew the mean. For example, if 19 of the six-year olds stand on one foot between 5 and 35 seconds, but one child stands for 180 seconds, the mean would be substantially higher than the 17 seconds and not represent the typical performance of the group. In general, when a test is standardized on a large number of children, one extreme score does not influence the result as dramatically as in this example because the other scores offset it.

Another measure of central tendency is the *mode.* This is the score that occurs more often than any other single score. For example, the modal age of first graders is six. In Table 1, the mode is 15 because this score occurs three times, whereas all the other scores occur only once or twice. The mode is often used with *nominal* or *categorical data* and when scores are so highly *skewed* that one value predominates.

A third measure of central tendency is the *median*. The median is the score most in the middle of all the scores. It is the point or score that divides the distribution of scores in half. In Table 1, the data is ranked from highest to lowest and the score in the middle (between the 10th and 11th scores of 17 and 15) is 16, thus the median is 16. The median is used when data are in *ranks*, or when the presence of a few extreme scores distorts the arithmetic average (the mean). It is the value of the median that is also its limitation. The median does not reflect the magnitude of the impact of every score in the distribution, even when certain of these scores are very high or very low. For example in Table 1, if one of the children, Daphne, had stood on one foot for 115 seconds instead of 19 seconds, the median of the distribution would not have changed and would continue to be reflective of the scores in the distribution. On the other hand, the mean would have changed from 17.2 to 22.0.

The mean, median, and mode are differentially related depending on the symmetry or skew of a distribution.[2] In some distributions (i.e., the normal curve, where the distribution is symmetric and unimodal), all three measures of central tendency are equal, but in many distributions they are different. The choice of which measure is best will differ from situation to situation. The mean is used most often because it includes information from all of the scores. However, when a distribution has a small number of very extreme scores, the median may better describe central tendency.[3]

Variability

Another method of describing a set of scores is by their *variability*, also known as *measures of dispersion*. For example, suppose it is known that the average six-year-old can stand on one foot for 17 seconds. Amanda however was only able to stand on one foot for 15 seconds. How can Amanda's performance be interpreted? What is normal for her age group? Knowing the average score helps but is not enough. The range of scores that are considered appropriate for a six-year-old needs to be considered. That is why variability is examined, to determine whether different groups of scores have different dispersions or distributions.

For example, in the following 2 sets of scores both have a mean of 3.

Set A: 1,2,2,3,3,3,4,4,5

Set B: 1,1,1,2,3,4,5,5,5

However, graphically it is obvious that they are very different (see Figure 1). If only indicators of central tendency were provided, the two sets of data would not be adequately described. An indicator of the variability or dispersion of the scores is necessary.

Two ways of describing the variability of a set of scores are in common use. The *range* is the difference between the largest and the smallest scores in a distribution. It is calculated by subtracting the smallest score from the largest score, and adding one. This measure is crude and unstable. As can be seen in the preceding example, the range $[(5\text{-}1) + (1) = 5]$ is the same for both sets of scores. Also, one high or low score would have a major effect on the range.

A more frequently used measure is the *variance*. This is a measure of the total amount of variability in a set of test scores. The variance is based on the difference between each individual's score and the mean of the group. The variance measures how widely the scores in a distribution are spread about the mean. It is calculated by subtracting the difference between each score and the mean, squar-

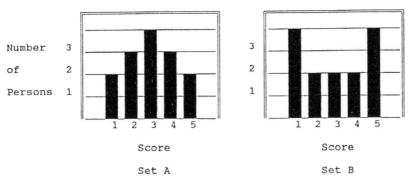

FIGURE 1. Distributions from Two Sets of Scores, Each with a Mean of 3

ing each of these numbers, adding them, and dividing the total sum of squares by the number of scores.[4]

Since the variance is calculated using squared deviations, the result is in terms of *squared units*. Because squared units are unwieldy to use in other calculations, generally the *square root of the variance* is computed. The square root of the variance is known as the *standard deviation*. It is the most commonly used measure of variability, and indicates the dispersion of scores around a given score, usually the mean. Generally, the larger the standard deviation, the more widely scattered are the scores. In the preceding example (Figure 1), the standard deviation of the scores in set A is 1.15 ($\sqrt{12/9}$) and in set B is 1.69 ($\sqrt{26/9}$). The importance and application of the standard deviation is discussed in the sections on normal curve and standard score.

The Normal Curve and Other Types of Distributions

The *normal curve* is a statistically derived distribution and is particularly helpful for comparing a child's score to that of other children. The *baseline* of the normal curve is divided into *whole and fractional standard deviation units* and serves as an interpretive yardstick for contrasting different examinee's test performances.

The normal curve is a *symmetrical bell-shaped curve*, in which the mean, median, and mode are identical. Because of the properties of the normal curve, the distribution can always be divided into predictable proportions, and there is an exact relationship between the area bounded by given standard deviation units and the proportion of cases found within that area under the curve (see Figure 2).

The total area under this curve equals 100%. Thirty-four percent of the cases (representing 34% of the area under the curve) are expected to fall between the mean and plus one standard deviation. Similarly, the area between the mean and minus one standard deviation represents 34% of the total area. It can be seen by examining Figure 2 that the area under the normal curve between plus and minus one standard deviation of the mean is 68%, thus if the sample is normally distributed, 68% of the cases would receive scores in this range. Furthermore, 95% of the area under the normal curve is

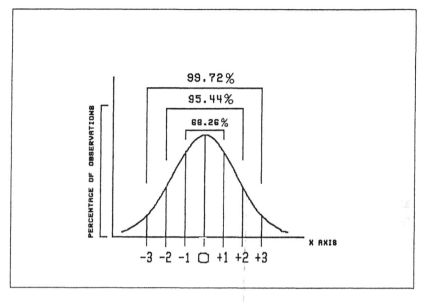

FIGURE 2. The Normal Curve

between plus and minus two standard deviations, and 99.7% of the area is between plus and minus three standard deviations.

Since the majority of scores are between −1.0 and +1.0 standard deviations from the mean (that is, 68% of the scores fall in this range), scores in this range are generally considered within normal limits. A standard score below −1.0 is considered to reflect possible dysfunction and a standard score above +1.0 is considered to represent a strength. (As discussed in Chapter 7, when interpreting an individual score, it is important to consider the standard error of measurement.)

Although many educational and behavioral variables are distributed in an approximately normal manner, not all scores fall into a normal distribution. On some measures, scores cluster at one end of the curve in what is known as a *skewed distribution.* For example, on the Space Visualization Contralateral Use (SVCU) score (derived from hand usage on the Space Visualization Test of the *Southern California Sensory Integration Tests*),[5] scores of seven-year-olds tended to cluster in the 26-29 range, although a few children obtained scores in the 0-25 range.[6] In this instance, when describing the average or typical performance of seven-year-olds, use of the group mean of 26 (and standard deviation of 3.8) would not be appropriate. The few low scores lowered the mean so that it did not reflect typical performance. Since the maximum score on the SVCU is 29, the few low scores could not be offset. In fact, a better measure of central tendency with this distribution is the mode (28), because it occurred more than twice as frequently as any other score, and thus is a better representation than the mean of what a "typical" seven-year-old would score.

Figure 3 shows the distribution of test scores for the 30 seven-year-olds in the study. This is a *negatively skewed distribution*.

Skew refers to the symmetry of a distribution. The distribution of scores on a test that is easy and on which most students earn high scores is known as a *negatively skewed distribution*. Conversely, on a very difficult test in which most children earn low scores, the distribution tails off to the higher end of the continuum and is called a *positively skewed distribution*. Figure 4 shows an example of a positively and negatively skewed distribution.

NORMS AND SCORES

One of the distinguishing characteristics of a standardized test is the provision of norms to aid in the interpretation of individual scores. Norm-referenced test interpretation involves some method of examining how an individual's test score compares to the scores of others in some known group. An individual's test performance is typically interpreted by comparing it to the performance of a group of subjects of known demographic characteristics (age, sex, race, etc.). This known group is called the *normative sample* or *norm group*. Norms are usually in the form of a table of equivalents between raw scores (i.e., number of correct responses) and one of several *derived scores*.

Derived scores are based on a transformation of the raw score to some other unit of measurement which enables comparison to the norm. One method of conceptualizing the kinds of *transformation* scores can undergo is by categorizing them as either *Developmental Scores* or *Within Group Measures*.[4] In developmental norms, the

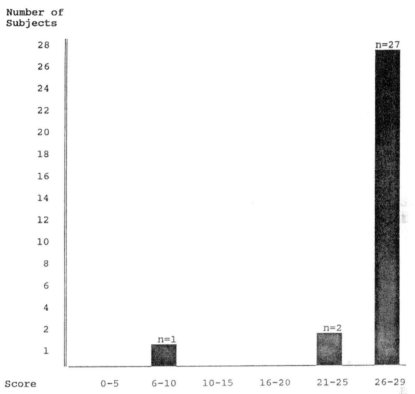

FIGURE 3. Negative Skew of the Distribution of Scores for Seven-Year-Olds on the SVCU

individual's performance is compared to the performance of children at many ages, and the score gives an indication of "how far along the normal developmental path the individual has progressed."[4,p77] In within group norms, the individual's score is compared to performance of a standardization group, usually of comparable age or grade. Whereas within group scores have a uniform and clearly defined quantitative meaning, developmental norms are psychometrically less sophisticated.[4] How test results are organized and presented depends to a large extent on the type of interpretation to be made. The various types of transformed scores are listed below,

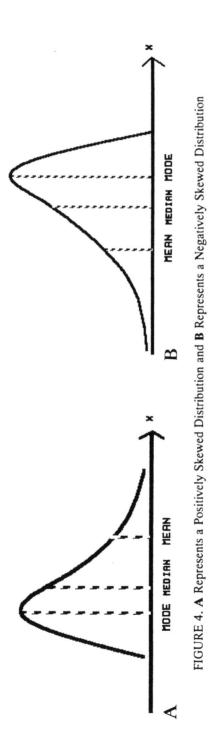

FIGURE 4. **A** Represents a Positively Skewed Distribution and **B** Represents a Negatively Skewed Distribution

grouped in the appropriate category. The following discussion examines each type of score within the two categories.

Developmental Scores	Within Group Scores
age equivalent	percentile rank
grade equivalent	standard scores
ordinal scale	stanines
	deviation IQs

Age Equivalent Scores

The *age equivalent* of a particular raw score is the chronological age of those children whose mean raw score is the same as the raw score in question; it is the raw score that a child at the 50th percentile in a particular age group would receive. The *Developmental Test of Visual-Motor Integration* (VMI)[7] is a test that uses age equivalents to report scores (although the more current revision of the test includes both age equivalents and a number of other methods to convert raw scores).[8]

For example, suppose that the average performance of 10-year-olds on the VMI was 17 correct drawings and that Michael drew 17 of the forms correctly. He would then have earned an age equivalent score of 10 years. Generally, age equivalents are expressed in years and months, using a hyphen.[2] For example, a score of 10 years 4 months is commonly represented by 10-4.

The primary advantage of age norms is that they are easily understood. However, many variables cannot be expressed meaningfully using age norms. For example, acuity of vision does not change during childhood. If a 20-year-old has 20/20 vision (which is normal for a 10-year-old also) it is not meaningful to say that the 20-year-old has an age equivalency score of 10-0. In addition, for many factors the age norms are only appropriate within a certain period of growth. For example, on a test of tactile perception, a 16-year-old might receive an age equivalent score of 8-0 because certain tactile perceptual abilities mature in the 6- to 8-year range (e.g., performance of a 6- to 8-year-old would be comparable to performance of an adult). If the score of the 16-year-old were written out in age equivalents as 8-0, it would appear as dysfunction, when in fact it represents normal abilities.

An additional problem with age equivalents is that a year's difference at one time in life is frequently different than a year's growth at another time. Take the example of a child who is delayed one year. If the child's chronological age is four and the child is delayed one year, this is a 25% delay because the age equivalency score (3) divided by the chronological age (4) is 75%. However, if the child is 10, and is delayed one year, his delay is only 10%, because the age equivalency score (9) divided by the chronological age (10) is 90%.

An additional problem with age equivalency scores is that they represent what a child in a particular age group at the 50th percentile would receive for a score. However, what is actually "normal" includes scores lower than the 50th percentile (in fact, performance as low as the 16th percentile which is one standard deviation below the mean is generally considered to be within normal limits). If there is a skewed distribution in the norm sample, the interpretation of age scores becomes even more difficult.

Grade Equivalent Scores

Grade norms or *grade equivalents* are often used in educational and academic achievement tests. A grade equivalency score means that a child's raw score is the average performance for that grade (grade equivalents may be based on the median or mean).[9] Thus, a grade equivalent of 4.6 is read as fourth grade, sixth month level. (The summer months are assumed to represent an increment of one month on the grade equivalent scale.)[9] Generally, a decimal point is used in the representation of grade scores.

The advantage of grade equivalency scores is that they are easy to understand. The disadvantages are similar to those presented for age equivalency scores in that they are easily misinterpreted. For example, Niki, a sixth grade child achieved a reading grade of 9.5 on the *Wide Range Achievement Test* (WRAT).[10] This does not mean that she reads at the ninth grade level. It means that what she knows as a sixth grader, she knows well. She did very well on a sixth grade reading test but did not take a ninth grade reading test.

Since grade equivalency scores depend on the particular items placed on a test and the particular norm group used, they are not interchangeable between tests or for different forms which are administered to different grades. It is a misinterpretation to say that a grade equivalent of 3.2 on the WRAT means the same thing as a grade equivalent of 3.2 on the *Peabody Individual Achievement Test*.[11] Also, grade equivalency scores between subtests, even on the same test, are not necessarily comparable.

Another problem with grade equivalency scores is that test publishers often do not have the financial resources to do a nationwide stratified sampling of children of all ages, grades K through 12, on a month-by-month basis. The publishers usually test at only a few grades, establish a relationship between test scores and grades, and then use the *relationship line* (a statistical manipulation) to estimate the various grade-month points.[9,12] These estimates are made by *interpolation* and *extrapolation*, and are often based on the assumption that what is tested is consistent from year to year. Nitko[9] provides further elaboration of the methodology in computing grade equivalents.

Another problem with the use of grade equivalency scores alone is that they do not provide information about an individual's percentile standing. Thus, an individual might get a higher grade equivalent on a reading test than on a mathematics test, yet have a substantially lower percentile rank on the reading test than on the math test.

Table 2 displays a hypothetical third grade pupil's test results. In Melissa's case, two identical grade equivalents have the same percentile rank. With Deborah, one grade equivalent can be higher than another yet associated with a lower percentile rank than the lower grade equivalent. This is because the scores for one subject area are more variable than for another.

Ordinal Scales

Ordinal scales, another type of developmental score, are based on developmental sequences, and are used to identify stages reached by a child. Qualitative descriptions are often provided. In ordinal scales, successful performance at one level implies successful performance at other preceding levels. The scales developed

TABLE 2. The Relationship Between Grade Equivalents and Percentile Ranks for Three Students

Child	Grade Equivalent	Percentile Rank	Grade Equivalent	Percentile Rank
Melissa	3.9	80	3.9	80
Sara	3.9	68	3.3	68
Deborah	3.9	68	3.6	74

within this framework are based on the sequential patterning and uniformity of developmental sequences. For example, in grasp, use of the entire hand in palmar prehension precedes thumb in opposition to the palm which precedes thumb-finger opposition.

An early example of the application of ordinal scales is the work of Gesell and associates[13] in which the sequential patterning of early behavior development is emphasized. The most well known ordinal scales are Piaget's stages of development.[14] These stages, which span the period from infancy through adolescence, are known as the sensorimotor, preoperational, concrete operational, and formal operational stages. Examples of ordinal scales based on the work of Piaget are the *Ordinal Scales of Psychological Development* designed for children ages two weeks to two years,[15] and the *Concept Assessment Kit-Conservation*, designed for ages four to seven years.[16]

Rank ordering of tasks is performed first in designing an ordinal scale, then age may be considered. Since these scales generally provide information about what the child is actually able to do, they share important features with criterion-referenced tests. A major problem encountered in ordinal scales is inconsistency in the anticipated sequences. "There is a growing body of data that casts doubt on the implied continuities and regularities of intellectual data."[17,p276] Moreover, when dealing with special populations, the developmental sequence may not be the same for the handicapped child as for the non-handicapped child.

Percentiles

A *percentile rank* indicates an individual child's position relative to the standardization sample. It represents the percentage of the standardization group who scored at or below a given raw score.[2,3,4,9] For example, if a raw score of 33 indicates a percentile rank of 80, it means that 80% of the group members had raw scores of 33 or less. Conversely, a student with a score of 33 scored as well as or better than 80% of the normative sample on the test.

The middle score in a distribution is the one that equals 50% of the scores. This score, at the 50th percentile, is the median and describes the average performance in a percentile distribution.[3]

A percentile-equivalency table typically provides raw scores and their percentile equivalents. The *Miller Assessment for Preschoolers* is an example of a test that utilizes percentiles.[18] The scoring system for the *Test of Motor Impairment* is also based on percentiles.[19] This test yields an index of dysfunction which is based on the percentage of subjects in the standardization sample scoring in a comparable manner.

Advantages of percentiles are that they are easy to understand, easy to compute, and suitable to any type of test. Therefore, they are widely adaptable and applicable. In addition, the table of norms can always be interpreted in the same way, regardless of the nature of the distribution of raw scores from which they are derived.[20] In other words, even when the distribution of scores is not normal, the interpretation of percentile norms does not change.

However, when using percentile ranks, it is important to remember that they refer to the percentage of persons earning equal or lower scores and not the percentage of items answered correctly. Also, percentile ranks do not increment equally with raw score intervals. In other words, if a change from the 50th to the 60th percentile represented an improvement of 5 raw score points, the change from the 85th to the 95th percentile would not also represent 5 raw score points if the scores are normally distributed. Since scores tend to be clustered near the middle in a normal distribution, a small raw score change near the center would result in a larger percentile change. A larger raw score difference at the extreme ends of the curve is needed to yield comparable percentile changes. This point is illustrated in Table 3 in performance on the *Stanford-Binet Intelligence Scale*[21] which has a mean of 100 and a standard deviation of 16.

As can be seen, an increase in 16 IQ points from 100 (the average score) to 116 represents a shift from the 50th to the 84th percentile, a change of 34 percentile units. In contrast, an increase in IQ of the same 16 points, but from a score of 132 to 148 (which is near the high end of the distribution), represents a percentile shift of less than two percent. Because of this characteristic of percentiles, these norms are ordinal not interval scales. As such, it is inappropriate to compute arithmetic means of these values or correlate them with other measures using a Pearson product-moment coefficient.[20]

Standard Scores

Standard scores express an individual's distance from the mean in terms of standard deviation or variability of the distribution. As previously described, a percentile only indicates how a specific individual's test score compares to other examinees from the standardization sample. However, a standard score represents in standard deviation units where an examinee's score is *with reference to the mean* of the distribution of the standardization sample.

TABLE 3. Relationship Between IQ and Percentile Scores

IQ Score	Percentile	% change
100	50	34
116	84	
132	98	14
148	99.9	2

Standard scores are derived scores that transform raw scores in such a way that the set of scores always has the same mean and the same standard deviation. They are used appropriately only with *equal-interval* or *ratio scores*. The advantages of standard scores are that they have uniform meaning from test to test and scores can be compared between tests. Moreover, unlike the percentile, the standard score unit has the same meaning throughout the range as illustrated in Table 4. As can be seen, an increase in IQ of 16 points (one standard deviation) from either 100 to 116, or from 116 to 132, or from 132 to 148 each represents a standard score increment of 1. In contrast, these score changes represent percentile rank changes of 34%, 14%, and 2% respectively. A disadvantage to standard scores is that they are not as familiar to the layperson.

There are several types of standard scores. Some of the most commonly used types are *z-scores*, *deviation IQ*, and *stanines*.

A z-score is defined as a standard score with a mean of 0 and a standard deviation of 1. A raw score is converted to a z-score using the equation:

$$z = \frac{X - \overline{X}}{SD}$$

In the equation, X = the raw score, $\overline{X}$ = the mean, and SD = the standard deviation.

Z-scores are interpreted in standard deviation units. Thus, a z-

TABLE 4. Relationship Between IQ, Percentile and Standard Scores

IQ Score	Standard score	Percentile	% change
100	0.0	50	34
116	1.0	84	
132	2.0	98	14
148	3.0	99.9	2

score of +1.5 means that the score is 1.5 standard deviations above the mean of the standardization sample. A z-score of −0.8 means that the score is .8 standard deviations below the mean.

Using the example presented previously of six-year-old Amanda who stood on one foot for 15 seconds will further explain this point. The average for the norm group was 17.3 seconds (see Table 1) and the standard deviation was 3.8 seconds. Amanda's standard score would be:

$$z = \frac{15 - 17.3}{3.8} = \frac{-2.3}{3.8} = -.6$$

This can be interpreted that Amanda's score is six-tenths of a standard deviation from the mean. The negative sign shows that the score is *below* the mean. A score is negative when the raw score is below the mean and positive when the raw score is at or above the mean.

Examples of tests which use this unit of measurement are the *Southern California Sensory Integration Tests*[22] and the *Sensory Integration and Praxis Tests.*[23] By using this form of scoring, it is possible to compare a score on one test to a score on another test, and to compare different subtests within a single test. In addition, when scores are distributed in a normal manner, z-scores can be converted to percentile scores. Table 5 provides a conversion of z-score to normal curve percentile rank correspondences. Using this table, Amanda's standard score (z-score) of −.6 would be equivalent to a percentile rank of 27.

A possible disadvantage to z-scores is that they contain decimals and minus values, which are sometimes confusing to interpret. Negative scores seem to imply a problem, however, any z-score between −1.0 standard deviations below the mean and +1.0 standard deviations above the mean is considered to be within normal limits.

In order to circumvent this possible misunderstanding, measurement specialists have developed a variety of scoring systems to transform z-scores, so that all scores within normal limits will be positive. The general procedure involves selecting a desired new mean and standard deviation. All z-scores are then multiplied by the

TABLE 5. Normalized z-Scores and Percentile Equivalents

z SCORE	PERCENTILE	z SCORE	PERCENTILE
3.0	99.9	-0.1	46.0
2.9	99.8	-0.2	42.1
2.8	99.7	-0.3	38.2
2.7	99.6	-0.4	34.5
2.6	99.5	-0.5	30.9
2.5	99.4	-0.6	27.4
2.4	99.2	-0.7	24.2
2.3	98.9	-0.8	21.2
2.2	98.6	-0.9	18.4
2.1	98.2	-1.0	15.9
2.0	97.7	-1.1	13.6
1.9	97.1	-1.2	11.5
1.8	96.4	-1.3	9.7
1.7	95.5	-1.4	8.2
1.6	94.5	-1.5	6.7
1.5	93.3	-1.6	5.5
1.4	91.9	-1.7	4.5
1.3	90.3	-1.8	3.6
1.2	88.5	-1.9	2.9
1.1	86.4	-2.0	2.3
1.0	84.1	-2.1	1.8
0.9	81.6	-2.2	1.4
0.8	78.8	-2.3	1.1
0.7	75.8	-2.4	0.8
0.6	72.6	-2.5	0.6
0.5	69.1	-2.6	0.5
0.4	65.5	-2.7	0.4
0.3	61.8	-2.8	0.3
0.2	57.9	-2.9	0.2
0.1	54.0	-3.0	0.1
0.0	50.0		

W.J. Popham, MODERN EDUCATIONAL MEASUREMENT, (c) 1981, p. 167. Reprinted by permission of Prentice-Hall, Inc., Englewood Cliffs, NJ.

new standard deviation followed by addition of the new mean. One example is known as the *T-score*. A T-score is simply a z-score multiplied by 10 (to eliminate the decimal) and with 50 added (to eliminate the minus value).[12] T-scores have a mean of 50 and a standard deviation of 10. An example of a test that uses T-scores is the *Walker Problem Behavior Checklist*,[24] a checklist of child behaviors and characteristics which is completed by the child's teacher and/or parent. Other commonly used derived scores have a mean of 100 and a standard deviation of 15 or 16.

Normalized Standard Scores

When scores fall in a normal distribution, it is possible to state precisely what proportion of the distribution's scores are exceeded by a score at a particular point along the baseline of the curve. For example, a raw score which is + 1 standard deviations above the mean in a normal distribution of scores equals or exceeds 84% of all the scores.

However, not all distributions are normal. When it is believed that the attribute being measured is normally distributed in the real world, but the data are distributed in a non-normal fashion, for ease of interpretation, the raw scores can be converted to *normalized standard scores*. A normalized standard score is a standard score (z or T) that would be equivalent to a raw score if the distribution had been normal.[12] The Standing Balance test of the *Southern California Sensory Integration Tests*[22] is an example where failure of the normative sample raw scores to assume a *bell-shaped curve* resulted in an alternate method of scoring standing balance. Non-linear transformations used to calculate normalized standard scores are further described in Popham.[12]

Deviation IQ Scores

One type of normalized standard score is the *deviation IQ score* used with certain tests of mental abilities such as *Wechsler Intelligence Scale for Children-Revised.*[25] The deviation IQ is actually a standard score with a mean of 100 and a standard deviation of 15. (Some IQ tests, such as the *Stanford-Binet Intelligence Scale,*[21] use a standard deviation of 16.) For example, if Bethany has an IQ of 115, this means she has scored one standard deviation above the mean for her age group (and has a percentile rank of 84).

The deviation IQ is valuable to control for variability caused by raw score distributions that have different standard deviations at different ages. The deviation IQ is only comparable from age to age or from test to test when using the same standard deviations. Wechsler was the first to use the deviation IQ in the *Wechsler Adult Intelligence Scale.*[26] The deviation IQ is also used in the revision of the *Stanford-Binet Intelligence Scale.*[21]

Stanines

A variation of the standard score is the *stanine scale* which is a system of derived scores that divides the distribution of raw scores into nine parts (the term stanine was derived from standard nines).[27] The highest stanine score is 9, the lowest is 1, and stanine 5 is located precisely in the center of the distribution. In normal distributions, stanines have a mean of 5 and a standard deviation equal to 2. Thus, a score between 3 to 7 stanines is considered within normal limits. The percentage of a group that falls within each stanine in a normal distribution is as follows:

Stanine	1	2	3	4	5	6	7	8	9
Percentage	4	7	12	17	20	17	12	7	4

One of the greatest advantages of stanines is that they can be applied to any type of data that approximate a normal distribution and that can be ranked from high to low. The top four percent of the students are assigned to a stanine of 9, the next seven percent to a stanine of 8, etc. Since an individual's stanine is determined by identifying the percentile to which a person's raw score would be equivalent, and then using the percentages to locate the proper stanine, stanines are a form of normalized scores.[12] For example, if Julio's score were equivalent to the 21st percentile, then his score would be in the third stanine.

Disadvantages to stanines are that they reflect coarse groupings of scores. However, this is seen as an advantage by some educators who, because of the imprecision of measurement "prefer to use gross descriptors in communicating test results and thus not misrepresent the precision of data-gathering devices."[12,p169] An example of a test that reports scores in stanines is the *Bruininks-Oseretsky Test of Motor Proficiency.*[28]

Relationship of Percentile, Standard Score, Normalized Standard Score, Deviation IQ (Types of Within Group Scores)

The relationship among stanines, percentiles, as well as other standard scores is shown in Figure 5.

If the scores are based on a normal distribution and when certain statistical conditions are met, then the different types of scales can be translated into any of the others.[4] However, it is important to use caution with between-test comparisons since variables such as the standardization samples may be different and an individual's relative standing on the tests may vary as a function of the standardization sample. For example, the normative sample for the *Screening Test for Auditory Comprehension of Language*[29] was composed of children from Tennessee, whereas the standardization sample for the *Southern California Sensory Integration Tests*[22] was from Los Angeles.

Interpreting Norm Scores

Table 6 provides a summary of various norm-referenced scores. Each type of score describes an individual's performance in reference to his/her location in a norm group. As discussed previously, each type of score has certain advantages and disadvantages. For example, grade-equivalents are easy to understand but are frequently misinterpreted. Standard scores are technically more accurate than grade-equivalents but are more difficult for the layperson to understand.

In considering norm scores, it is important to recognize that they provide relative rather than absolute information. Norms reflect how a particular group (the norm group) performed on a particular test at a particular point in time. Norms as such should not be considered as performance "standards." By nature of the type of scores, 50% of scores are below the mean, and 50% are above the mean. It does not make sense to consider bringing all subjects "up to normal." Similarly, norm scores do not provide any information about the mastery of a skill, although it is often assumed that if a score is greater than −1.0 standard deviations below the mean, then performance is within normal limits and therefore acceptable.

SUMMARY AND RECOMMENDATIONS

Raw scores, or the number of correct or incorrect answers that a child obtains on a test provides the examiner with relatively little information. In order to be meaningful, raw scores must be converted to a type of reference system. Norm-referenced interpretation is a relative interpretation which is based on the individual's position with respect to some group, usually called the normative group.[3] Two types of norm-referenced comparisons can be made, across ages and within ages. Developmental scores such as age equivalents and grade equivalents compare the performance of students across ages or grades. Within age (or within group) comparisons can be made using several different types of scores such as stanines, standard scores, etc., each with certain advantages and disadvantages.

The manuals accompanying standardized tests should contain tables that permit a tester to convert raw scores to various derived scores such a percentile ranks or standard scores. Some tests such as the *Bruininks-Oseretsky Test of Motor Proficiency*[28] or the *Developmental Test of Visual-Motor Integration*[8] provide one set of tables for converting raw scores to percentiles, and another set of tables for converting to age equivalents. Table 7 presents a list of types of scores provided by tests commonly used by occupational and physical therapists.

The selection of the particular type of score to use and to report depends on the purpose of testing and the sophistication of the consumer. Salvia and Ysseldyke[2] recommend against the use of developmental scores because they are readily misinterpreted. Percentile ranks have the advantages that (a) they require the fewest assumptions for accurate interpretation, (b) the scale of measurement can be ordinal, equal-interval, or ratio data, and the distribution of scores need not be normal, and (c) they are readily understood.[2] Standard scores are convenient for test authors since their use allows the author to give equal weight to various subtests. Standard

FIGURE 5. Percentage of Cases Under Portions of the Normal Curve

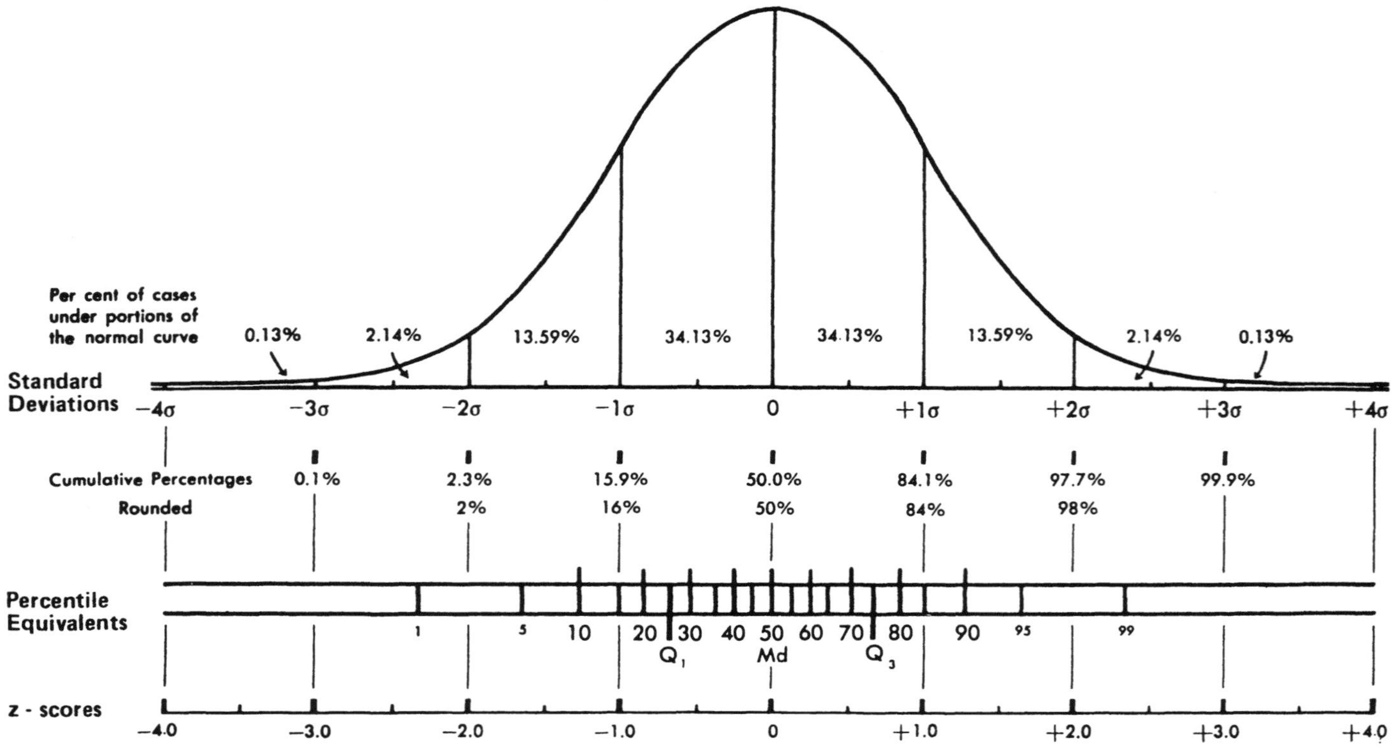

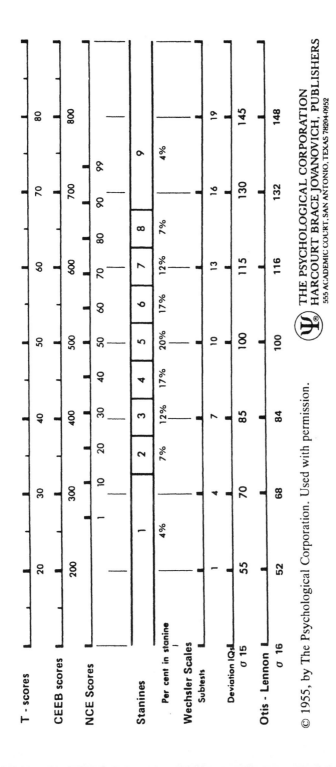

T - scores
20 · 30 · 40 · 50 · 60 · 70 · 80

CEEB scores
200 · 300 · 400 · 500 · 600 · 700 · 800

NCE Scores
1 · 10 · 20 · 30 · 40 · 50 · 60 · 70 · 80 · 90 · 99

Stanines
1 · 2 · 3 · 4 · 5 · 6 · 7 · 8 · 9

Per cent in stanine
4% · 7% · 12% · 17% · 20% · 17% · 12% · 7% · 4%

Wechsler Scales
Subtests
1 · 4 · 7 · 10 · 13 · 16 · 19

Deviation IQs
σ 15
55 · 70 · 85 · 100 · 115 · 130 · 145

Otis - Lennon
σ 16
52 · 68 · 84 · 100 · 116 · 132 · 148

THE PSYCHOLOGICAL CORPORATION
HARCOURT BRACE JOVANOVICH, PUBLISHERS
555 ACADEMIC COURT, SAN ANTONIO, TEXAS 78204-0952

TABLE 6. Summary of Various Norm-Referenced Scores

Type of Score	Interpretation	Score	Examples of Interpretations
Percentile Rank	Percentage of scores in a distribution at or below this point.	PR = 60	"60% of the raw scores are at or lower than this score."
z-Score	Number of standard deviation units a score is above (or below) the mean of a given distribution.	z = +1.5	"This raw score is located 1.5 standard deviations above the mean."
		z = -1.2	"This raw score is located 1.2 standard deviations below the mean."
Stanine	Location of a score in a specific segment of a normal distribution of scores.	Stanine=5	"This raw score is located in the middle 20% of a normal distribution of scores."
		Stanine=9	"This raw score is located in the top 4% of a normal distribution of scores."

Score	Definition	Example	Interpretation
Deviation IQ	Location of a score in a normal distribution having a mean of 100 and a standard deviation of 16.	IQ = 124	"This raw score is located 1.5 standard deviations above the mean in a normal distribution whose mean is 100 and whose standard deviation is 16. This score has a percentile rank of 93."
		IQ = 84	"This raw score is located 1.0 standard deviations below the mean in a normal distribution whose mean is 100 and whose standard deviation is 16. This score has a percentile rank of 16."
Grade-Equivalent Score	The grade placement at which the raw score is average.	GE = 3.5	"This raw score is the obtained or estimated average for pupils whose grade placement is at the 5th month of the third grade."
Age-Equivalent Score	The age at which the raw score is average.	AE = 7-6	"This raw score is the average score for students whose age is 7 years 6 months."

Adapted from Nitko[9,p.341]

TABLE 7. Types of Scores for Tests Commonly Used by Occupational and Physical Therapists

Type of Score

Test Names	Age Equi-valency	Standard Score	Percentile	Stanine	Other
Bayley Scales of Infant Development 1		*			
Peabody Developmental Motor Scales 30	*	*	*		
Denver Developmental Screening Test 31					*
Miller Assessment for Preschoolers 18			*		
Bruininks Oseretsky Test of Motor Proficiency 28	*	*	*	*	

Test of Motor Impairment [19]		*
Test of Visual Motor Integration–Revised [7]	*	* *
Southern California Sensory Integration Tests [22]		*
Sensory Integration and Praxis Tests [23]		*

scores are useful for the examiner since if the distribution is normal, they can be converted to percentile ranks, and also can be used in profile analysis. According to Anastasi,[4] standard scores are the most satisfactory type of derived score. At the stage that decisions are being made about scoring systems by test developers, it is critical to employ experts in tests and measurements as consultants.

REFERENCES

1. Bayley N: *Bayley Scales of Infant Development*. New York, Psychological Corporation, 1969.

2. Salvia J, Ysseldyke JE: *Assessment in Special and Remedial Education*. Boston, Houghton Mifflin, 1985.

3. Wiersma W, Jurs SG: *Educational Measurement and Testing*. Boston, Allyn & Bacon Inc, 1985.

4. Anastasi A: *Psychological Testing*, ed 6. New York, Collier Macmillan Publishers, 1988.

5. Ayres AJ: *Interpreting the Southern California Sensory Integration Tests*. Los Angeles, Western Psychological Services, 1976.

6. Cermak S, Quintero J, Cohen P: Developmental age trends in crossing the body midline in normal children. *Am J Occp Ther.* 34:313-319, 1980.

7. Beery KE: *Developmental Test of Visual-Motor Integration, Administration and Scoring Manual*. Chicago, Follett Publishing Company, 1967.

8. Beery KE: *Revised Administration, Scoring, and Teaching Manual for the Developmental Test of Visual-Motor Integration*. Cleveland, Modern Curriculum Press, 1980.

9. Nitko, AJ: *Educational Tests and Measurement: An Introduction*. New York, Harcourt Brace Jovanovich, 1983.

10. Jastak JF, Jastak SR: *WRAT Manual: The Wide Range Achievement Test*. Wilmington, DE, Guidance Associates of Delaware, 1965.

11. Dunn LM, Markwardt FC: *Peabody Individual Achievement Test*. Circle Pines, MN, American Guidance Services Inc, 1970.

12. Popham WJ: *Modern Educational Measurement*. Englewood Cliffs, NJ, Prentice-Hall, 1981.

13. Gesell A, Amatruda CS: *Developmental Diagnosis*, ed 2. New York, Hoeber-Harper, 1947.

14. Piaget J: *The Origins of Intelligence in Children*. New York, International Universities Press, 1952.

15. Uzgiris IC, Hunt J: *Assessment in Infancy: Ordinal Scales of Psychological Development*. Urbana, University of Illinois Press, 1975.

16. Goldschmid ML, Bentler PM: *Manual: Concept Assessment Kit-Conservation*. San Diego, Educational and Industrial Testing Service, 1968.

17. Anastasi A: *Psychological Testing*, ed 5. New York, Macmillan Publishing Co Inc, 1982.

18. Miller LJ: *Miller Assessment for Preschoolers*. San Antonio, TX, Psychological Corporation, 1988, 1982.

19. Stott DH, Moyes FA, Henderson SE: *Test of Motor Impairment, Henderson Revision*. Guelph, Ontario, Brook Educational Publishing Ltd, 1984.

20. Ahmann JS, Glock MD: *Evaluating Student Progress*, ed 6. Boston, Allyn & Bacon Inc, 1981.

21. Thordike RL, Hagen EP, Sattler JM: *Stanford Binet Intelligence Scale*, ed 4. Chicago, Riverside Publishing Co, 1986.

22. Ayres AJ: *Southern California Sensory Integration Tests Revised*. Los Angeles, Western Psychological Services, 1980.

23. Ayres AJ: *Sensory Integration and Praxis Tests*. Los Angeles, Western Psychological Services, in press.

24. Walker HM: *Walker Problem Behavior Identification Checklist*. Los Angeles, Western Psychological Services, 1983.

25. Wechsler D: *Wechsler Intelligence Scales for Children-Revised*. New York, Psychological Corporation, 1974.

26. Wechsler, D: *Wechsler Adult Intelligence Scale-Revised*. New York, Psychological Corporation, 1981.

27. Grolund NE: *Measurement and Evaluation in Teaching*. New York, Macmillan, 1985.

28. Bruininks RH: *Bruininks-Oseretsky Test of Motor Proficiency, Examiner's Manual*. Circle Pines, MN, American Guidance Service, 1978.

29. Carrow E: *Screening Test for Auditory Comprehension of Language*. Austin, TX, Learning Concepts, 1973.

30. Folio MR, Fewell RR: *Peabody Developmental Motor Scales and Activity Cards Manual*. New York, Teaching Resources Corporation, 1983.

31. Frankenburg WK, Dodds JB, Fandal AW, Kazuk E, Cohrs M: *Denver Developmental Screening Test, Reference Manual*, rev ed. Denver, CO, LaDoca, 1975.

KEY POINTS

1. A norm-referenced standardized test provides norms to aid in the interpretation of individual scores.

2. A group of test performance scores can be described by examining measures of central tendency where one number (mean, median, or mode) represents the performance of the group.

3. A group of test performance scores can also be described by their variability (range or variance) which indicates whether

different groups of scores have different dispersions or distributions.

4. The normal curve is a symmetrical bell-shaped curve in which the mean, median, and mode are identical, and the distribution can always be divided into predictable proportions.

5. Derived scores are based on a transformation of the raw scores to some other unit of measurement which enables comparison to the norm.

6. Age scores are easily understood. A disadvantage is that many variables cannot be expressed meaningfully, because for many factors age norms are only appropriate within a certain period of growth. Age scores represent what a child at the 50th percentile would receive for a score (although "normal" includes lower scores).

7. Grade equivalency scores mean that a child's raw score is the average performance for that grade. They are easy to understand but have disadvantages similar to age equivalency scores.

8. Ordinal scales, a type of developmental score, are based on developmental sequences and are used to identify stages reached by a child. A major problem with them is that successful performance at one level implies successful performance at other preceding levels.

9. Percentile rank indicates an individual child's position relative to the standardization sample. Advantages include that they are easy to understand, compute, suitable to any type of test, and widely adaptable and applicable. However percentile ranks do not increment according to raw score value; therefore means cannot be calculated and they cannot be used to calculate correlations.

10. Standard scores express an individual's distance from the mean in terms of standard deviation or variability of the distribution. Raw scores are transformed in such a way that the set of scores always has the same mean and the same standard deviation. Their primary advantages are that they have uniform meaning from test to test and scores can be compared between tests. Their main disadvantage is lack of familiarity to laypersons.

11. A disadvantage of z-scores (a type of standard score) is that

they contain decimals and minus values which are sometimes confusing to interpret. T-scores can transform the z-scores so that all scores within normal limits are positive.

12. The stanine is a system of standard scores that divides the distribution of raw scores into nine parts. Stanines can be applied to any type of data that approximate a normal distribution and can be ranked from high to low. The primary disadvantage is that they reflect coarse groupings of scores.

13. It is important to use caution with between-test comparisons of scores since variables such as the standardization samples may be different and an individual's relative standing on the tests may vary as a function of the standardization sample.

14. Norm scores provide relative rather than absolute information. Norms reflect how a particular group (the norm group) performed and should not be considered as performance "standards."

15. Selection of the type of scores to use and report depends on the purpose of testing, sophistication of the intended users, and the types of interpretations to be made.

Chapter 6

Reliability

Jean C. Deitz

You can prove almost anything with the evidence of a small
enough segment of time. How often, in any search for truth,
the answer of the minute is positive, the answer of the hour
qualified, the answers of the year contradictory!

—Edwin Way Teale
"January 6," Circle of the Seasons (1953)

INTRODUCTION

One of the primary concerns of the occupational or physical therapist who is developing a test is the *reliability* of the instrument s/he
is constructing. Reliability concerns the consistency of test scores
and the extent to which measurements are repeatable when different
persons make the measurements, on different occasions, and using
different instruments that are intended to measure the same construct. This type of information is essential for validating clinical
judgments that are based on test scores.

A test score actually consists of two different scores: the *true
score* and the *error score*.[1] A person's true score is his/her test score
unaffected by chance factors. The true score is a hypothetical construct. If the person always obtained the same score even when the
examiner and internal and external testing conditions were varied,
that score would be the person's true score. In reality, this never

Jean C. Deitz, PhD, OTR/L, FAOTA, is Assistant Professor of Rehabilitation
Medicine at the University of Washington, Seattle, WA 98195.

happens. All measurement on a continuous scale has a component of error. No test is completely reliable. Reliability is always a matter of degree. *Measurement error* is associated with a variety of factors. Some of the more common include lack of agreement among scorers, inconsistent performance among examinees, failure of an instrument to measure consistently, and failure of the tester to follow standardized testing procedures.

Measures of reliability indicate the amount of measurement error in a set of scores. As the error component increases, the amount of confidence a therapist can have in the obtained test scores decreases. Basically, the reliability of a test depends on two factors. The first is the amount of measurement error and the second is the ability of the test to discriminate among differing levels of ability within the group being tested. According to Baumgartner and Jackson, acceptable reliability can be achieved when the subjects, the test, the testing environment, and the examiner meet certain criteria.[2] It is preferable that participants in reliability research be ". . . heterogeneous in ability, motivated to do well, ready to be tested, and informed about the nature of the test."[2,p99] Baumgartner and Jackson also have summarized other factors that are conducive to reliability: (1) power to discriminate among ability groups; (2) sufficient length so that each subject can show his or her best performance without being penalized for an unrepresentative poor trial; (3) test organization designed to optimize examinee performance; and (4) test administration and scoring instructions that are clear and precise. In addition, the testing environment should support good performance and the examiner should be competent in administering the test.[2] For tests designed to be appropriate for a wide age range, reliability should be examined for each age level and not for the group as a whole.[3]

TYPES OF RELIABILITY

As Feldt and McKee point out, "there is no single index which may be rightfully called the reliability of the test."[4,p281] The test developer must identify which factors of the many influencing the obtained score are due to true differences in the characteristics under consideration and which are due to chance errors.[4] Then, on the basis of this information, s/he must decide which types of reliability are most appropriate to the purpose and characteristics of the test being developed.

Once the test developer has designed a reliability study, s/he must determine the optimal sample size for the study. Often, in the early stages of test development, pilot reliability studies are conducted with samples of 10 to 15 subjects. However, studies designed for publication in test manuals and journal articles typically have 20 or more subjects. Optimal sample size is influenced by the purpose of the reliability study, the type or types of reliability examined, the characteristics of the sample, and the characteristics of the statistic employed as an index of reliability. Ideally, sample sizes should be determined before beginning the study and in consultation with a statistician.

Four basic types of reliability are traditionally reported in test manuals. They are *test-retest reliability, interrater reliability, alternate-forms reliability*, and *internal consistency estimates of reliability*. In most cases, estimates of reliability are obtained by correlating test scores. Hence, the *reliability coefficient* is usually expressed as a value between 0 and 1, with higher values indicating higher reliability. The use of correlational methods is described in greater detail later in this chapter in the section on statistics.

Test-Retest Reliability

Test-retest reliability refers to the stability of test scores over time. Stability is extremely important for tests that are to be used clinically and which should not be appreciably affected by repetition. A therapist cannot have confidence in a client's scores if they change from one testing session to the next. Test-retest reliability indicates the extent to which test scores are stable over time and the degree to which they are subject to the random daily changes in the client, the examiner, the environment, and the test instrument. To assess test-retest reliability, the same test is administered to the same individuals on two separate occasions; the scores obtained on the first and second administrations of the test are then compared. For example, the manual for the *Bruininks-Oseretsky Test of Motor Proficiency* reports a test-retest reliability study that was conducted with a sample of 63 second graders and 63 sixth graders.[5] The children were tested twice within a seven to twelve day period. Reliability coefficients for each subtest, fine and gross motor composites, and the short form of the test were reported for each of the two age categories. In studies such as this, it is important that variables such as the testing conditions and the tester be held constant.

When designing a test-retest reliability study, a test developer must make several decisions. First, the *time interval* between test and retest should be determined. As a general rule, the longer the interval between testings, the lower the reliability.[6] Currier maintains that there should be enough time between test administrations to "reduce or prevent the effects of memory, practice, and transfer effects of contact with other respondents."[7,p150] Anastasi warns against too much time between test and retest and states that "for any type of person, the interval between test and retest should rarely exceed six months."[1,p110] She adds that shorter intervals between test and retest are appropriate with infants and young children for whom discernible developmental changes can be expected within a limited time frame. Obviously, this same consideration should be used in designing a test-retest reliability study for any client population for whom changes may occur within a short time due to a disease process or expected course of recovery. Baumgartner and Jackson maintain that test-retest reliability is probably the most appropriate type of reliability for physical performance measures since psychomotor learning is less apt to vary within a time span of one or two days. They suggest a test-retest interval of one to three days for most physical measures, and a seven-day interval for maximum effort tests where fatigue is involved.[2] In summary, the time interval between test and retest varies according to the age of the examinees and the type of test and should be chosen to minimize the effects of memory, practice, and development on test scores.

Second, in designing a test-retest reliability study, the test developer should consider examiners' levels of expertise. Finally, the test developer must make decisions about the standardization of the test and retest environment and how much latitude will be allowed relative to the time of day testing is to take place. Ideally, the time of day for the test and retest should be the same.

Interrater Reliability

Interrater or interscorer reliability refers to the consistency of test scores when they are determined by different examiners. The examination of this type of reliability is particularly important for tests that depend largely on the examiner's judgment. It relates to the *error variance* that reflects the amount or degree of agreement between examiners.[8]

Interrater reliability involves a comparison of the scores obtained by two or more examiners who independently score or rate the performance of each subject. For example, in assessing interrater reliability for the *Miller Assessment for Preschooler* (MAP), Miller used two raters.[8] One field supervisor administered the MAP to a child and scored it while another observed and independently scored the performance of the same child. Each field supervisor administered the MAP to 20 children. The scores of the two field supervisors were compared for the total MAP and for each of the five subtests. This study is an example of a common design for assessing interrater reliability. It can be expanded to include more raters or it can be designed to include examination of reliability for separate age groups or disability groups.

Before conducting interrater reliability research, the test developer can take steps to help insure good interrater reliability for the test. The first is to include detailed instructions in the test manual regarding test administration and scoring procedures. The test developer should then subject these to review, both by experts in the area of testing and clinicians who are unfamiliar with the test but who are potential users. On the basis of their feedback, the administration instructions should be revised. Next, the revised instructions should be tried out on another small group of clinicians who also are unfamiliar with the test but are potential users. The test administration and scoring of this group should be evaluated. Procedural inconsistencies should be noted and the instructions in the test manual should be modified accordingly. Steps in this process can be repeated until the test developer is confident that the test administration and scoring instructions are complete, clear, and objective and that it is feasible for clinicians to make the types of judgments the test requires them to make. This preliminary work will help to insure good interrater reliability.

The next step is to design and conduct a formal interrater reliability study. Examiners who participate in the study should be similar to those for whom the test is intended.[9] For example, if the test manual states that the test can be administered by occupational therapists and aides, interrater reliability should be examined for both of these groups and not just occupational therapists. Also, the type and amount of training provided to the examiners should be clearly specified. If the results are to be generalizable to the clinic setting and training is required, the clinician should have an opportunity to acquire similar training. For example, if it is essential that the test developer individually train the examiners, this would lead to a highly restricted use of the test. If, on the other hand, video training tapes are developed and used to prepare testers for the interrater reliability study, these tapes can be distributed as part of the test manual. Similarly, if a training module that includes competency tests is used to prepare testers for the reliability study, these materials also can be made available to the clinician. In other words, if raters for a reliability study are trained, comparable training opportunities should be available for potential test users.

Alternate-Form Reliability

Alternate-form reliability refers to the consistency of test scores for two forms of the same test. *Equivalent* or *parallel forms* are tests measuring the same thing at the same level of difficulty, so that equal raw scores have the same meaning on each form. Obviously, this type of reliability can only be determined by means of parallel forms, each form consisting of a unique set of items.

In order to assess alternate-form reliability, two forms of the same test typically are administered approximately two weeks apart in order to allow for the occurrence of variations in attitude and ability.[9] It is further recommended that the research design counterbalance the order of presentation. Given two forms of a test, Form A and Form B, half of the subjects would complete Form A first and half of the subjects would complete Form B first.

Alternate-form reliability is useful if a person must be tested twice and a learning or practice effect is expected. It is particularly important when one form of the test will be used as a pretest and a second form will be used as a posttest.[3] A primary benefit of alternate-form reliability, identified in the *Standards for Educational and Psychological Tests* is that it eliminates memory as a systematic source of variance.[3] As Anastasi points out, this type of reliability also reduces the impact of *practice effects*.[1] However, she warns that it will not eliminate them. Alternate-form reliability is still influenced by error due to differences in item content, subjectivity of scoring, and variability in people's performance over short periods of time.

To date, due to the stage of occupational and physical therapy in relation to testing, no tests designed specifically for the therapy fields have alternate forms. Examples of alternate-form reliability can be found in test manuals for various achievement and cognitive tests.

Internal Consistency Estimates of Reliability

Internal consistency estimates of reliability relate to the homogeneity of test items. They describe how well all of the items measure the same variable,[10] or in a multiple trial test, the consistency of performance from trial to trial.[2] According to Currier, this type of reliability is used when "construction of an alternate or equivalent form of the instrument is not feasible," or when having two or more administrations of the same instrument is unwise.[7,p155] For example, memory and experience with the test could be expected to influence an examinee's scores on a test involving problem-solving skills. Internal consistency estimates of reliability are more appropriate for relatively long tests with many items.

Two primary methods can be used to determine an internal consistency estimate of reliability. The first method is referred to as the *split-half technique*. It involves correlating scores obtained on one half of the test with those obtained on the other half of the test. The result is an estimate of reliability based on a test which is only half the length of the original test. The *Spearman-Brown formula* is used to correct for this reduction in test length.[11]

Several approaches have been used to divide a test into two

equivalent halves. One of the most common is the odd-even split where alternate items are placed in opposite halves of the test. Anastasi advises that when groups of items dealing with a single problem occur, all of the items in the group should be assigned to the same half of the test.[1] A second approach for dividing a test in half is to place alternate groups of items in each half of the test. A third method is to select pairs of items on the basis of equivalence in content and difficulty, and randomly assign one item in each pair to each half of the test. Thus, the test developer planning to use split-half reliability has several options for dividing a test into two equivalent halves. In making this decisions s/he should be guided by an awareness of the need to have each half of the test conform to the specifications of the total test.[6]

The second statistic that provides an internal consistency estimate of reliability is *coefficient alpha*. This statistic is based on the "average correlation among items within a test and the number of items[12,p333] and is used for tests that have multiple-scored items.[1] According to Nunnally, coefficient alpha is the first estimate of reliability that should be obtained, and if coefficient alpha is very low, either the test is too short or the items have little in common with each other.[9] In either case, revision of the test is indicated.

The *Kuder-Richardson technique* is a special version of coefficient alpha which is used with *dichotomous data*. The Kuder-Richardson reliability coefficient is "the mean of all split-half coefficients resulting from different splittings of a test."[1,p116] According to Anastasi, the "difference between Kuder-Richardson and split-half reliability coefficients may serve as a rough index of the heterogeneity of the test."[1,p116] This is because all possible splits are examined rather than one split chosen so that both halves contain equivalent sets of items.

The American Psychological Association has warned against treating estimates of internal consistency as substitutes for other types of reliability.[3] Chance errors are more likely to affect the scores on both halves of the same test and this results in a tendency toward inflated estimates of reliability.

Baumgartner and Jackson suggest that test-retest reliability coefficients are better indicators of reliability for psychomotor tests and warns that internal consistency estimates of reliability are not appropriate for maximum performance tests.[2] For example, consider a test of grip strength involving four trials using a vigorimeter. If the sample consisted of children with arthritis, it is likely that fatigue would be a factor and that a decreasing pattern of grip strength scores with each successive trial would be noted. This could lower the internal consistency estimate of reliability since, with this method, change in scores from trial to trial is viewed as measurement error.

Aspects to Be Included in the Written Reports

Once reliability studies are completed, the test developer should report the results and details of the studies in the test manual or a technical report. Specific information to be provided includes: rationale for selecting the type of reliability studied, brief rationale for selecting a time interval (test-retest and alternate studies), interval between administrations (test-retest and alternate studies), design of the study, data collection procedures, characteristics of the data collectors, characteristics and size of the sample (age, sex, etc.), type of analysis used, actual reliability coefficients, qualifications and training of testers or raters, and conditions under which the test was administered. This information must be provided so that potential test users can evaluate the results of the reliability studies and know to whom and under what conditions the results are likely to generalize.

Standard Error of Measurement

The *standard error of measurement* (SEM) provides an estimate of the amount of variation expected in an individual's test score across repeated measurements, and it is useful in interpreting a test score for one individual. The SEM indicates the limits within which an individual's test scores are expected to vary due to measurement error. According to Baumgartner and Jackson, it "acts like a test score's standard deviation, and can be interpreted in much the same way using the normal curve."[2,p98] For example, the person's observed score plus or minus one standard error of measurement will equal the range of the person's true score approximately 68% of the time, while the person's observed score plus or minus two standard errors of measurement will equal the range of the person's true score approximately 95% of the time. According to Nunnally, the size of the standard error of measurement is a direct indication of the amount of error involved in using a particular instrument.[9] It is directly related to the reliability coefficient. The smaller the reliability coefficient, the larger the standard error of measurement and the less confidence there can be in the obtained test score.

One method of calculating the standard error of measurement is to take the square root of the quantity one minus the reliability coefficient and multiply this quantity by the standard deviation of a set of test scores.[1]

$$SEM = (SD) \sqrt{1 - r}$$

The reliability coefficient used in this formula usually is that of alternate forms or test-retest reliability, rather than intertester reliability. The standard error of measurement is directly related to the magnitude of the standard deviation of the test.[6] Thus, when comparing two different tests, their standard errors of measurement should be evaluated in light of the magnitudes of their respective standard deviations.[6] (See Horn for a discussion of other methods of calculating the standard error of measurement.)[13]

In addition to reporting the standard error of measurement in the test manual, test developers in occupational and physical therapy should consider developing score sheets so that test scores are reported with *confidence bands*. For example, consider a test with a total possible score of 20 for each of two subtests, one for fine motor and one for gross motor. Each subtest has a standard error of measurement of 1. The hypothetical client received a score of 10 on the fine motor subtest and a score of 8 on the gross motor subtest. If confidence bands of plus or minus one standard error of measurement were used, this client's scores would be reported as they appear in Figure 1. If approximately 95% confidence was desired this client's scores and confidence bands for plus or minus two standard errors of measurement could be reported (see Figure 2).

Reporting test scores by using confidence bands helps to emphasize the element of error in all measurement. It provides a concrete representation of the amount of confidence a test user can have concerning an individual's test score.

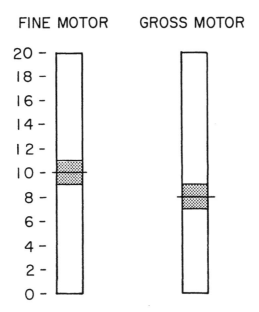

FIGURE 1. Using Confidence Bands to Report Test Scores (68% Confidence Interval)

DESIGNING RELIABILITY RESEARCH FOR A TEST

Understanding the various types of reliability and their respective purposes can help the test developer design the reliability research for the test. Then, the test developer should consider all factors that could produce measurement error of concern relative to the purpose and use of the test. Next, since it is neither technically nor practically possible to incorporate all of these in the design of the study or studies, the test developer must determine which of these factors are most important. For example, consider a test of fine-motor skills for four-year-old children. Potential influences on a child's scores that a test developer might want to study include the tester, the day, and the time of day. This would require the examination of both interrater reliability and test-retest reliability. Since both day-to-day fluctuations and time-of-day fluctuations in scores were identified as potential sources of error, the reliability research should be designed to address these. In addition, all relevant variables should be

FINE MOTOR   GROSS MOTOR

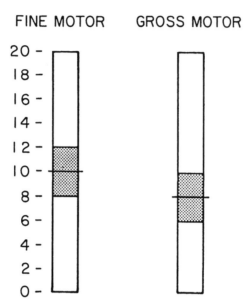

FIGURE 2. Using Confidence Bands to Report Test Scores (95% Confidence Interval)

counterbalanced. Figure 3 is an example of such a design for examining interrater and test-retest reliability in which it is possible to study the effects of time of day, examiner influences, and sex of subject.

As can be seen in Figure 3, each tester serves as test administrator for half of the boys and half of the girls and as scorer for the other half of the subjects. Ideally, the testers should alternate the role of test administrator. In addition, in the retest situation, the therapist who initially tested the child, retests the child seven days later. Also, half of the children are retested at the same time of day and half of the children are retested at the opposite time of day.

Such a study is resource and time effective in that the original test data for the interscorer reliability study are used in the examination of test-retest and internal consistency reliability. In addition, designs of this type facilitate the examination of the extent and interrelationships of various sources of measurement error. Using such an approach, each potential influence on scores can be examined as an experimental variable and a more comprehensive picture of the reliability of the test can be obtained. For additional information, refer to writings on generalizability theory.[13,14]

STATISTICS

A variety of statistics have been used as measures of reliability. Test developers are confronted with choosing the statistics most suited to the design of their study, the type of data with which they are dealing, and the particular questions they are tying to answer.

Pearson Product-Moment Correlation Coefficients

Traditionally, when the data are interval or ratio and score distributions are approximately normal, one of the most common statistics used for calculating reliability is the *Pearson product-moment correlation coefficient*. It has been used for interrater reliability, test-retest reliability, parallel form reliability, and split-half reliability. Relative to the latter, it should be noted that once the correlation between the two halves of the test is determined, the Pearson product-moment correlation coefficient is entered into the *Spearman-Brown prophecy formula* in order to determine reliability for the full test.[1]

The Pearson product-moment correlation coefficient expresses the degree of relationship between two variables. Both Nunnally and Shelley agree that when this statistic is employed, an index of reliability of .90 is the minimum standard for measures used for clinical purposes.[9,12] They further agree on .80 as an acceptable standard for basic research purposes. In contrast, Benson and Clark indicate that .60 or greater is acceptable for test-retest reliability and .80 or greater is acceptable for parallel form reliability.[16]

Currently, there is controversy over the use and meaning of the Pearson product-moment correlation coefficient as an expression of the degree of reliability.[17] Some authors cite this statistic as the primary statistic used to determine the reliability of an instrument, [1,16,18] but other authors question its use.[2,6,7]

The Pearson product-moment correlation coefficient compares changes in group rankings from one set of measures to the next.

FIGURE 3. Sample Plan for Conducting Reliability Studies (Note 1: In the initial test situation, using a stratified random approach, subjects would be assigned to Therapist A or Therapist B and to either morning or afternoon test sessions. Note 2: Scores from the initial test administration to 40 boys and 40 girls could be used when examining internal consistency reliability.)

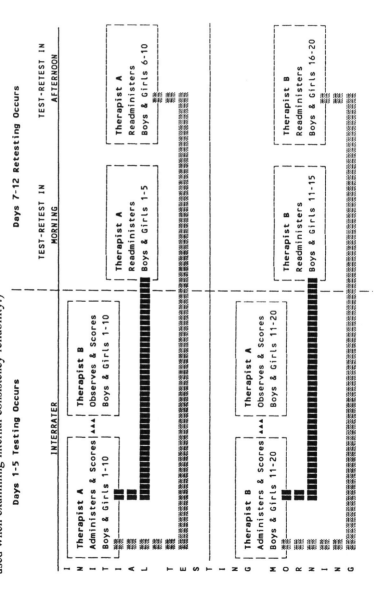

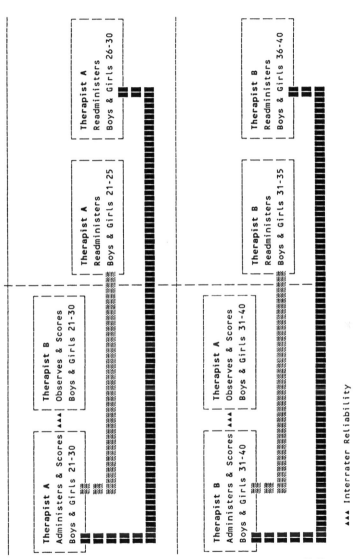

However, it does not compare absolute change in scores between two sets of measures. Consider a test-retest reliability situation in which each patient earned exactly the same score on the test and the retest. Using the Pearson product-moment correlation coefficient, this would be an example of perfect test-retest reliability. However, the situation in Table 1 also exemplifies perfect reliability even though each subject's score doubled on the retest.

This occurs because in the calculation of the Pearson product-moment correlation coefficient, each score is converted to a standard score and then the relationship between these scores is determined. This conversion is necessary because the Pearson product-moment correlation coefficient is designed for use in bivariate situations where the relationship between two sets of scores, each from a different test, is to be determined.[6] This makes it possible to compare scores from two different tests such as the *Bruininks-Oseretsky Test of Motor Proficiency*[5] and the *Peabody Developmental Motor Scales*.[19] However, the method of calculation used allows systematic changes such as those exemplified in Table 2 to go undetected.

Table 1

An Example of Scoring Patterns Which Result in Perfect Test-Retest Reliability Using the Pearson Product-Moment Correlation Coefficient

	Test	Retest
Subject A	1	2
Subject B	2	4
Subject C	3	6
Subject D	4	8
Subject E	5	10

Table 2

Types of Reliability and Their Corresponding Statistics

Type of Reliability	Level of Measurement	Statistic Employed
Test-Retest and Alternate Form Reliability	Interval or Ratio*	Pearson Product-Moment Correlation Coefficient
		Intraclass Correlation Coefficient
	Ordinal	Spearman Rank Correlation Coefficient
		Kendall Rank Correlation Coefficient
Interrater Reliability	Interval or Ratio*	Pearson Product-Moment Correlation Coefficient
		Intraclass Correlation Coefficient
	Ordinal	Spearman Rank Correlation Coefficient
		Kendall Rank Correlation Coefficient
		Kendall's Coefficient of Concordance

TABLE 2 (continued)

Type of Reliability	Level of Measurement	Statistic Employed
Internal Consistency	Interval, ratio or Ordinal	Coefficient Alpha
	Dichotomous	Kuder-Richardson
Internal Consistency (Split-Half)	Interval or Ratio*	Pearson Product-Moment Correlation Coefficient and Spearman-Brown Prophecy Formula
	Ordinal	Spearman Rank Correlation Coefficient and Spearman-Brown Prophecy Formula
		Kendall Rank Correlation Coefficient and Spearman-Brown Prophecy Formula

* Approximately normal score distributions required

Therefore, at a minimum, if this statistic is employed, score distributions should be examined for systematic changes. These will be reflected either by significant differences between the means or the variances of the two distributions. In addition, a scatterplot of the two sets of scores can be created and examined.

Another limitation of this statistic, as well as its nonparametric analogues, is that it can only be used when there is a maximum of two raters or two trials. This greatly restricts designs for reliability studies.

Intraclass Correlation Coefficients

In view of the limitations of the Pearson product-moment correlation coefficient, numerous authors advocate the use of the *intraclass correlation coefficient* for determining test-retest reliability, interrater reliability, and alternate form reliability.[2,4,20-22] This statistic provides an estimate of test reliability that is a correlation coefficient derived from analysis of variance.[2] Unlike the Pearson product-moment correlation coefficient, the intraclass correlation coefficient is based on a univariate distribution (i.e., the distribution of a single variable, as when there are repeated measurements of children on the same test). However, like the Pearson product-moment correlation coefficient, it is only appropriate for use with continuous data that are approximately normally distributed.

Baumgartner and Jackson enumerated several benefits of the intraclass correlation coefficient.[2] First, it can be used whether scores are collected on one day or several days. Second, it allows for more than two scores per person, for more than two raters, or for one rater over several trials. Third, it is sensitive to more sources of measurement error. Fourth, it is the only method that considers changes in the mean and standard deviation from one set of measures to the next to be measurement error.

For example, consider an interrater reliability study where Rater A consistently scored higher than Rater B. In such a situation, the mean score of Rater A would be higher than that of Rater B even if they ranked the subjects similarly. This difference in scoring would be reflected in the magnitude of the intraclass correlation coefficient.

When the intraclass correlation coefficient is used for calculating interrater reliability, raters are entered into the formula as trials.[2] Examples of interrater reliability studies using intraclass correlation coefficients can be found in the literature. Kielhofner, Harlan, Bauer, and Maurer used intraclass correlation coefficients to examine the interrater reliability of two examiners in rating a historical interview.[23] Hanten and Pace used intraclass correlation coefficients to examine the reliability of measuring anterior laxity of the knee joint using a knee ligament arthrometer.[24]

Like the Pearson product-moment correlation coefficient, the magnitude of the intraclass correlation coefficient is influenced by the homogeneity of the sample for the reliability study. When the group is highly homogeneous, the result is a small sum of squares among subjects which in turn results in a lower intraclass correlation.[2] When this occurs, one of the best ways to improve the reliability of the test is to increase the sensitivity of the test relative to the population for whom it is designed.

Shrout and Fleiss point out that different versions of the intraclass correlation coefficient give different results even when applied to the same data.[18] Because of this they advocate that the investigator report the **exact form** of the intraclass correlation coefficient used in the reliability study. These authors also provide specific guidelines for researchers using intraclass correlation coefficients.[21] Other writers provide additional examples and formulas for intraclass correlation coefficients.[2,20,21,22,25] (See Table 2 for further information regarding statistics employed for the various types of reliability.)

SUMMARY AND RECOMMENDATIONS

When examining reliability, the test developer must decide what sources of measurement error are of concern for the test and then design studies accordingly. In doing this, the test developer should obtain data from natural groups comparable to the expected test examinees. For tests designed to be appropriate for a wide age range, reliability should be examined for each age level separately. Due to the characteristics of most statistics used as indices of reliability, the latter will result in inflated estimates of reliability.

Also, the test developer must remember that reliability is a prerequisite to validity, but it does not insure validity. A test may be a reliable measure and still be an invalid measure of that which it is intended to measure. Even so, the importance of reliability should not be underestimated. As Kerlinger says, "High reliability is no guarantee of good scientific results, but there can be no good scientific results without reliability."[26,p455]

REFERENCES

1. Anastasi A: *Psychological Testing*. New York, MacMillan Publishing Co, 1988.

2. Baumgartner T, Jackson AS: *Measurement for Evaluation in Physical Education and Exercise Science*. Dubuque, IA, Wm C Brown Publishers, 1987.

3. American Psychological Association: *Standards for Educational & Psychological Tests*. Washington DC, American Psychological Association, 1974.

4. Feldt LS, McKee ME: Estimation of reliability of skill tests. *Res Quart* 29(3): 279-293, 1958.

5. Bruininks RH: *Bruininks-Oseretsky Test of Motor Proficiency*. Circle Pines, MN, American Guidance Service, 1978.

6. Safrit M: *Evaluation in Physical Education*. Englewood Cliffs, NJ, Prentice-Hall Inc, 1973.

7. Currier D: *Elements of Research in Physical Therapy*. Baltimore, Williams & Wilkins Co, 1979.

8. Miller LJ: *Miller Assessment for Preschoolers*. San Antonio, TX, Psychological Corporation, 1988, 1982.

9. Nunnally J: *Psychometric Theory*. New York, McGraw-Hill Book Co, 1978.

10. Tuckman BW: *Conducting Educational Research*. New York, Harcourt Brace Jovanovich Inc, 1978.

11. Ebel RL, Frisbie D: *Essentials of Educational Measurement*. Englewood Cliffs, NJ, Prentice-Hall Inc, 1986.

12. Shelly SI: *Research Methods in Nursing and Health*. Boston, Little Brown & Co, 1984.

13. Horn CJ: Integration of concepts of reliability and standard error or measurement. *Educ Psychol Measmt* 31:57-74, 1971.

14. Cronbach LJ: *Essentials of Psychological Testing*. New York, Harper & Row, 1984.

15. Cronbach LJ Glesser GC, Nanda H, Rajartnam N: *The Dependability of Behavior Measurements*. New York, Wiley & Sons, 1972.

16. Benson J, Clark F: A guide for instrument development and validation. *Am J Occup Ther* 36(12):789-800, 1982.

17. Michels E: Measurement in physical therapy. *Phys Ther* 63(2): 209-215, 1983.

18. Payton O: *Research: The Validation of Clinical Practice*. Philadelphia, FA Davis Co, 1979.

19. Folio MR, Fewell RR: *Peabody Developmental Motor Scales*. Allen, TX, Developmental Learning Materials Teaching Resources, 1983.

20. Bartko J: The intraclass correlation coefficient as a measure of reliability. *Psychol Rep* 19:3-11, 1966.

21. Shrout PE, Fleiss J: Intraclass correlations: Uses in assessing rater reliability. *Psychological Bulletin* 86(2):420-428, 1979.

22. Lahey MA, Downey RG, Saal FE: Intraclass correlations: There's more there than meets the eye. *Psychol Bull* 93(3):586-595, 1983.

23. Kielhofner G. Harlan B, Bauer D, Maurer P: The reliability of a historical interview with physically disabled respondents. *Am J Occup Ther* 40(8):551-556, 1936.

24. Hanten WP, Pace MB: Reliability of measuring anterior laxity of the knee joint using a knee ligament arthrometer. *Phys Ther* 67(3):357-359, 1987.

25. Winer BJ: *Statistical Principles in Experimental Design*. New York, Mc-Graw-Hill, 1962.

26. Kerlinger FN: *Foundations of Behavioral Research*. New York, Holt Rinehart & Winston Inc, 1973.

KEY POINTS

1. Reliability concerns the consistency of test scores and test administration. Reliability is a matter of degree and depends on the amount of measurement error.

2. Test-retest reliability refers to the stability of test scores over time. The time interval between test and retest varies according to the age of the examinees and the type of test.

3. Interrater reliability refers to the consistency of test scores when they are determined by different examiners. Two or more examiners independently score or rate the performance of each subject and then compare the scores obtained.

4. If raters for a reliability study are specifically trained, comparable training opportunities should be available for potential test users.

5. Alternate-form reliability refers to the consistency of test scores for two forms of the same test which measure the same thing at the same level of difficulty. This type of reliability is useful if a person must be tested twice and a learning or practice effect is expected.

6. Internal consistency estimates of reliability relate to the homo-

geneity of test items. They can be determined using the statistical methods of either the split-half technique or coefficient alpha. The Kuder-Richardson technique is a version of coefficient alpha for use with dichotomous data.

7. Standard error of measurement indicates the limits within which an individual's test scores are expected to vary due to measurement error. The smaller the reliability coefficient, the larger the standard error of measurement and the less confidence there can be in the obtained test score.

8. The test developer should carefully consider all factors that could produce measurement error, relative to the purpose and use of the test. After determining which of these factors are most important reliability studies can be designed.

9. When data are interval or ratio and score distributions are approximately normal, the Pearson product-moment correlation coefficient is the most common statistic used for calculating reliability. This coefficient expresses the degree of relationship between two variables and compares changes in group position from one set of measures to the next.

10. Limitations of the Pearson product-moment correlation include: systematic changes go undetected and it can only be used when there is a maximum of two raters or two trials.

11. Benefits of the intraclass correlation coefficient include: it can be used if scores are collected over several days; it allows for more than two scores, two raters, and for several trials; it is sensitive to more sources of measurement error; and it is the only method that considers changes in the mean and standard deviation from one set of measures to the next to be measurement error.

12. For tests designed for a wide range, reliability needs to be examined for each age level rather than the group as a whole.

13. Reliability is a *prerequisite to validity*, but it does not insure validity.

Chapter 7

Validity

Winnie W. Dunn

If you can't prove what you want to prove, demonstrate something else and pretend that they are the same thing. In the daze
that follows the collision of statistics with the human mind,
hardly anybody will notice the difference.

—Darrell Huff
How to Lie with Statistics *(1954)*

INTRODUCTION

The development of valid assessment tools is a high priority in
the allied health professions. Clinical assessment is a significant
aspect of the practice of occupational and physical therapy. Information gathered by means of clinical assessment provides a basis
for determining the need for intervention, remediation required, ef-

Winnie W. Dunn, PhD, OTR, FAOTA, is Associate Professor and Chairper-
son in the Occupational Therapy Education Department at the University of Kansas, Kansas University Medical Center, 39th & Rainbow Blvd., Kansas City, KS
66103.

The author would like to acknowledge Bonnie Danley for expert assistance in
manuscript preparation.

The editor would like to acknowledge Dr. Dunn's contributions to many of the
other chapters in this book. Because validity is a *process* of accumulating data
which verifies various aspects of the test, many pages of Dr. Dunn's original
manuscript were adapted into previous chapters: Chapter 2, operational definitions, table of specifications, and item selection; and Chapter 3, testing conditions. The editor appreciates the author's flexibility in allowing parts of her manuscript to be used elsewhere which greatly enhanced the quality of the total book.

149

ficacy of rehabilitation outcomes, and the client's prognosis. Assessment typically involves a complex process of problem solving and decision making. Since the therapist will ultimately be making important decisions about the patient's future, the clinical data upon which these decisions are based must be both comprehensive and accurate.

Although subjective and qualitative data (e.g., structured interviews and skilled observations) are valuable, clinical assessments frequently involve structured procedures or testing. The most important consideration in evaluating and selecting an assessment tool is its validity. Validity refers to the extent to which a test measures what it purports to measure. "The concept refers to the appropriateness, meaningfulness, and usefulness of the specific inferences made from test scores."[1,p9] Evidence of validity is essential for determining the usefulness of a test for a particular application.

Although the term "validity" has a commonsense meaning, the concepts underlying this meaning are not always evident. Professionals may be able to define validity and distinguish different types of validity theoretically. However, the practical application of these concepts in everyday therapeutic situations is more difficult. The purpose of this chapter is to outline a framework in which therapists can conceptualize the validation process for norm-referenced tests. It should be noted that in a work of this scope it is impossible to fully address the issue of validity. Rather, an overview of the processes is presented to provide basic information. Numerous references are noted which provide more comprehensive information about the types of validity.

VALIDITY IN THERAPEUTIC PRACTICE

In the course of practice, therapists may be faced with situations in which the process of clinical evaluation is inadequate to ascertain the client's problem or to formulate specific interventions. In these situations, commonly used clinical tests are either adapted or extended or the therapist is forced to design new techniques of measuring the observed problems. Assessment techniques which do not yield useful information are abandoned or modified for possible future applications. The diagnostic approach is usually based on the therapist's own previous professional experience.

This process is replicated in interpreting data from standardized tests. Valid and effective test use is directly related to the tester's expertise. The therapist's skilled observations provide additional important diagnostic information which may not be tapped through a given battery of tests. With experience, the therapist becomes better able to evaluate a wide range of problems. On the other hand, impressions that do not refer to objective and standardized criteria are often not sensitive to any but the grossest deficits in certain areas of functioning.[2]

Over years, a therapist's diagnostic skills are likely to evolve considerably as a result of ongoing refinements in both assessment procedures and professional judgment. Through this process, both evaluation and treatment skills are strengthened. This ongoing process results in the *validation of therapeutic practice*.

A similar process is undertaken in determining the validity of tests and assessment techniques. However, rather than relying on professional experience, the process involves formal and systematic studies which utilize agreed-upon conventions of data collection, analysis, and documentation. Formal methods of validation provide a basis for the interpretation of test results and evidence that is acceptable to professionals in other fields. Before an objective, standardized assessment can be used with confidence, its psychometric properties and therapeutic utility should be evaluated in detail and from different professional perspectives.

BASIC ISSUES IN VALIDITY RESEARCH

A Continuous Process

Validity is an elusive concept. It is not concrete, and thus cannot be directly observed, palpated or measured. Rather, it is inferred from research findings and applied experience using personal as well as generally accepted standards. An instrument's validity is dependent upon a number of factors, including the population or sample for which it is used, its internal properties, and its relationship to other variables.[1,3] Consequently, validity is initially investigated as an instrument is being developed, and confirmed through subsequent use.

Campbell and Stanley emphasize the continuous nature of validity research, which consists of replication and cross-validation.[3] These two types of research build a body of knowledge, and can increase confidence in the validity and usefulness of an instrument. Clearly, evidence of validity is accumulated knowledge and cannot be obtained from the results of a single investigation.

Responsibilities of the Test Developer and User

The test developer is initially responsible for providing potential users with adequate information to judge whether the test is appropriate for specific purposes and for a targeted clinical population. The *Standards for Educational and Psychological Testing* of the American Psychological Association (APA) states that "No test is valid for all purposes in all situations or for all groups of individuals. Any study of test validity is pertinent to only a few of the possible uses or inferences from the test scores."[1,p31]

It is the obligation of the test developer to provide cautions about inappropriate use of the test instrument. In circumstances where a test is to be used with a population dissimilar to the standardization sample, or in a situation significantly different than the one the test was validated in, it is the responsibility of the test user to validate the instrument.[1] Responsible use of test instruments rests in the hands of the users, though initial validity questions should be answered by the test developer.

The test developer is also responsible for providing normative data for an assessment tool. Since most instruments measure the presence of or deviation from a normal range of scores, the range of normal and abnormal performance must be clearly defined. Without this information, interpretation of test results is difficult or impossible.

Validation for Special Populations

Recent research has addressed questions related to the appropriateness of test instruments for special populations. Fuchs, Fuchs, Benowitz, and Barringer have noted that, as a result of important legislation, tests used to identify handicaps must now be validated for their intended use.[4] Following a review of widely used norm-referenced tests, these authors concluded that most test developers and publishers still provide little information concerning the appropriateness of specific tests with handicapped children. Due to qualitative differences in the functioning of special populations, assumptions of validity regarding test results for one group may not hold true for another group.

Fuchs et al. cite several studies which indicate that speech and language handicapped children perform less well with unfamiliar than familiar examiners.[4] No such effect was observed for nonhandicapped children. In this area, examiner familiarity has the effect of invalidating diagnostic and intervention decisions. *Cross-validation* studies are needed to rule out these kinds of systematic sources of error that may influence test results for different diagnostic subgroups.

In norming a test, it may be necessary to consider possible differences in the performance of subgroups. For example, recent research indicates that different normative criteria should be used to evaluate the performance of males and females on some tests of equilibrium.[2]

TYPES OF VALIDITY STUDIES

Evidence of validity for an assessment tool should answer two questions. First, what can an examiner infer about what is being measured by this test? Second, what might be inferred about other behaviors from the results of this test?[1]

The "ultimate validity" of a test can never be proven. Rather, ongoing use of an instrument contributes to accumulated evidence of validity. However, the relative validity of a test can be judged on the basis of several accepted categories. For example APA's *Standards for Educational and Psychological Testing* divides the types of validity into three categories: *content validity, criterion-referenced validity,* and *construct validity,* each of which is detailed below.[1]

Content Validity

Content validity is the degree to which test items represent the performance domain the test is intended to measure. Content validity can be established in a variety of ways including expert judgments, and certain logical and empirical procedures. The most important, initial task of test developers is to adequately describe the content of the test, and its proposed uses. One common method for specifying test content and organizing specific objectives is the development of a Table of Specifications (described in Chapter 2). Using sound, comprehensive methodology and a good panel of experts at this stage is essential to ensuring content validity.

Some authors discuss *face validity*[5,6] although the 1985 APA *Standards for Educational and Psychological Testing* does not consider this a specific standard.[1] Face validity refers to the ability of the test instrument to measure what it appears to measure. When designing items, test developers may survey a panel of experts regarding the existing item pool to determine which ones have good face validity.[5] For example, when designing an instrument to test various types of sensory processing, a group of experts might be asked to judge the items that have been designed according to the major sensation which is tapped.

Content validity also refers to the ability of the test instrument to *represent the universe of possibilities* for that area of function. For example, if the goal is to develop a comprehensive measure of fine motor performance, and only two items are selected, both requiring pincer grasps but not other forms of prehension, the test instrument may be judged as having poor content validity.

Content validity is usually determined through an examination of the relationship between test objectives and test items. Generally a panel of experts are used to assist in making this comparison. Moore suggests that there are two primary methods for obtaining professional opinions about the content validity of an instrument.[5] The first is to provide the panel of experts with the items from the test and request a determination of what the battery of items is measuring. The second method requires providing not only the test items, but also a list of the test objectives so that the experts can determine the relationship between the test items and the objectives.

Content validity is not indicated by a statistical measure but rather is inferred from these types of judgments.

The APA 1977 *Standards for Educational and Psychological Tests* contrasts content and face validity: "Content validity is determined by a set of operations and one evaluates content validity by the thoroughness and care with which these operations have been conducted. In contrast, face validity is a judgment that the requirements of a test merely *appear* to be relevant."[7,p29]

Clearly, content validity requires that the test developer provide a clear description of the domains addressed by the instrument. This is the only way that a test user can determine the applicability of the test for use in specific situations. For example, Gardner reports that content validity was established for the *Test of Visual Perceptual Skills* (TVPS),[8] through a process of identifying a comprehensive list of factors in visual perception, and then constructing items which represented these factors. Because Gardner[8] does not report use of the expert review procedures suggested by Moore[5] to assess content validity, the reader is left with an incomplete understanding of the process.

Criterion-Referenced Validity

Criterion-referenced validity refers to the ability of a test to systematically demonstrate a relationship to external criteria. Criterion-referenced validity may be demonstrated by concurrent or predictive studies. *Concurrent validity* is obtained by correlating two or more measures given to the same subjects at approximately the same time. *Predictive validity* is obtained by comparing a subject's performance at the initial time of testing, to performance obtained at a later date on another measure.

Concurrent Validity

Beery reports the results of concurrent studies using the *Developmental Test of Visual-Motor Integration-Revised* (VMI)[9] and the *Primary Mental Abilities Test* (PMA).[10] Interestingly, the relationship between these two measures was found to decrease with age (correlations of .59 for first graders, .37 for fourth graders, and .38 for seventh graders). Miller[11] evaluated the concurrent validity of the *Miller Assessment for Preschoolers* (MAP) in relation to measures of current developmental status including the *Wechsler Preschool and Primary Scale of Intelligence* (WPPSI),[12] *Illinois Test of Psycholinguistic Abilities* (ITPA),[13] *Southern California Sensory Integration Tests*,[14] and *Denver Developmental Screening Test*.[15] The author states,

> There is no single test so similar to the MAP that test scores for both could be directly compared with the expectation that there would be a direct positive correlation. It was anticipated that certain standardized tests would correlate with specific MAP performance indices, but no correlation would exist between MAP Total Score and the standardized test.[11,p109]

Specific findings for each of the concurrent validity studies are presented in the MAP manual. The author appropriately cautions that in absence of follow-up predictive validity data, the concurrent validity data are incomplete.

Predictive Validity

Predictive studies evaluate the relationship of the test to follow-up measures. For example, the predictive validity of a preschool screening test may be evaluated by relating screening outcomes to later school performance. Due to large individual differences in development, this type of validity is difficult to establish, particularly for young children. The test developer must also be able to track the same subjects from the initial testing to the later time period when the risk factors might become manifest. Interdependent relationships are difficult to sort out for measurement.

Predictive studies are valuable for a variety of purposes. For example, the test user may be able to evaluate an individual and forecast future job performance, determine potential future adjustment, or predict success when placed in a specified group. Researchers who have ''captive audiences'' over a period of time are in a better position to establish the predictive validity of a test instrument, and are less likely to have to contend with attrition.

Screening programs are dependent upon the predictive efficiency of test instruments.[16] Unfortunately, use of existing instruments often entails substantial risks of incorrectly identifying children. For example, errors can occur in identifying a child as handicapped when in fact there is no handicap, and in not identifying a handicapped child because the test is not sufficiently sensitive to deficits. Problems with predictive validity should cause test users to be cautious in instrument selection for screening programs.

Predictive validity methodology has evolved towards *classificational analysis* as a means for expressing predictive efficiency of instruments. This methodology allows for the comparison of accurate to inaccurate predictions and the calculation of several critical proportions which assign meaning to the validity of the predictive measure. Individual cases are analyzed relative to their inclusion into one of four categories.[17] *True positives* and *true negatives* occur, for instance, when the classification of subjects into "problem" or "no problem" groups, based on initial test results, is later confirmed by results on the criterion measure. *False positives* or *overreferrals* are cases classfied as "problem" yet no problem is revealed on the criterion. *False negatives* or *underreferrals* are cases classified as "no problem" who later have a "problem" as revealed on the criterion. The test developer strives to keep both false positives and false negatives to a minimum. Extensive discussion of classificational methodology is available in the research literature.[18,19,20]

Predictive validity studies often test hypotheses which are based on theoretical reasoning about relationships between variables. For example, some studies examine the relationship of motor abnormalities to later school performance.[21] To provide meaningful tests of this hypothesis, predictive validity studies involving scoring cutpoints and categories should include a sufficient sample. Since prediction falls into one of the four categories described above, testing five subjects would not be useful. Keppel suggests that sample size determination is dependent on the complexity of the research design.[22] In addition, when a series of tests are used, subjects would need to take them in different order; that will therefore mean that even more subjects will be required to cover all options in the design. Although there are formulas to assist researchers in determining sample size, Keppel acknowledges the difficulty in using them because the researcher must be able to predict anticipated outcomes to make use of them. Stangler, Huber and Routh provide an excellent work sheet to assist in calculating the various statistics used in classificational analysis[16] (see Table 1).

Criteria for membership in each outcome category should be established on an *a priori* basis before initiation of the study. Specifically, the level of performance which will lead to a classification of "problem," and the level of performance that will lead to a conclusion of "no problem," should be clearly defined. Careful planning helps the study run more smoothly, and leads to more meaningful results.

An example of a comprehensive predictive validity study is provided by Miller.[11] Four years after the MAP was originally administered during the standardization, approximately 25% of the original sample were relocated, and were assessed on a four-hour battery of tests including the *Wechsler Intelligence Scale for Children-Revised*,[23] *Woodcock-Johnson Psychoeducational Battery, Bruininks-Oseretsky Test of Motor Proficiency*,[25] *Goodenough-Harris Drawing Test*,[26] and Developmental Test of Visual-Motor Integration.[9] In addition, the follow-up criteria included six performance measures (i.e., retained in school, teachers' observations, report card grades, etc.). Both correlational and classificational methodology were employed to analyze the data. In summary, Miller found that the MAP total score consistently showed significant correlations with criterion measures, significant t-test differences between the mean scores of problem and no problem groups, and excellent classificational accuracy.[11] These findings were consistent across all standardized instruments, and all six school performance criteria. These findings provide accumulated evidence of the predictive validity of the MAP.

Construct Validity

Construct validity is "the extent to which a particular test can be shown to measure a hypothetical construct."[27,p281] The APA *Standards for Educational and Psychological Testing* emphasize that a test author must provide detailed information about the constructs upon which a test is based so that test users can determine the appropriateness of the test for populations that they serve.[1] Construct

Table 1

Worksheet for Calculating Screening Test Validity

		Criterion Test Results	
		Abnormal	Normal
Screening Test Results	Refer (positive)	a Correct referrals	b Incorrect referrals
	Do Not Refer (negative)	c Incorrect nonreferrals	d Correct nonreferrals

Rate of referral
$$= \frac{a + b}{a + b + c + d} \times 100$$

Rate of overreferral from total sample
$$= \frac{b}{a + b + c + d} \times 100$$

Rate of underreferral from total sample
$$= \frac{c}{a + b + c + d} \times 100$$

True Positives = a

False Positives = b

False Negatives = c

True Negatives = d

validity is a more abstract concept than the other types of validity discussed. It refers to the *underlying theoretical* premises and concepts that are measured by test scores. Moore regards construct validity as the broadest type of validity which encompasses all other types of validity.[5]

The construct validity of the test is originated in the planning phase and executed throughout the development of the test. Evidence of validity has its beginnings in the test developer's review of the literature. The decisions regarding the purpose of the test, exact constructs to be measured, operational definitions, item selection and administration procedures, and design of the development and standardization processes all affect the construct validity of the final product. Thus the methodology used to implement all aspects described in Chapters 2 through 6 have an impact on the test's construct validity.

Construct validity should be obtained whenever a test purports to measure an abstract trait or theoretical characteristics about the nature of human behavior. Examples of constructs provided in the literature include intelligence, self-concept, anxiety, school readiness, and perceptual organization. The five following areas must be considered in the validation of constructs with test instruments.[28,29]

1. Age Differentiation

Developmental change is a major consideration for tests designed to evaluate children. Although sensitivity to age trends is not the only evidence which should be provided, if it can be shown that test scores demonstrate a progressive increase corresponding to age, this will add to the accumulated evidence of the construct validity of tests for children.

2. Factor Analytic Study

Factor analysis is a statistical procedure which can assist in determining whether there are several theoretical domains within the same test. Factor analysis "simplifies the description of behavior by reducing the number of categories from an initial multiplicity of test variables to a few common factors, or traits."[28,p116] The procedure groups variables that are moderately or highly correlated with one another. Then the actual dimensions underlying the data can be compared with the construct design to determine whether the data support the hypothesized constructs.

For example, the results of factor analytic studies on the *Southern California Sensory Integration Test Battery* (SCSIT)[14] supported the various types of dysfunction the test was designed to identify. The *Kaufman Assessment Battery for Children* (K-ABC),[30] an intelligence test, reports two types of factor analytic research. Factor analysis was conducted for the Mental Processing Subtest alone, and for all subtests at each year of age. *Principal factor analysis* was used to illuminate the abilities underlying the set of tests, since the traits had not previously been identified. *Confirmatory factor analysis* was used more frequently in validating the K-ABC because most of the items had already been organized into scales. Results confirmed Kaufman's dichotomy into Sequential-Simultaneous for all ages; the Sequential-Simultaneous-Achievement construct differentiation was also confirmed for all ages.[30]

Factor analytic research for the *Bruininks-Oseretsky Test of Motor Proficiency* (BOTMP) revealed that the largest factor was a general motor development factor.[25] Many of the fine motor and several of the gross motor items clustered on this factor. Other factors only partially matched the test developer's organization of the subtest items. For example, subtest 3, Bilateral Coordination, has eight items on the test protocol, suggesting that these behaviors are homogeneous and represent a similar construct. However, factor analysis did not confirm the homogeneity of these items, since these eight items loaded on three different factors. Perhaps a conclusion of Bilateral Coordination as being a single construct is not warranted. This study indicates that further research would be valuable in this area.

It is also of interest to examine the factor structure of a test for different populations to ensure that the internal structure of a test does not differ among diagnostic subgroups. For example, a recent study reported by Meisels, Cross, and Plunkett[31] replicated for premature infants the factor structure of the Infant Behavior Record of the *Bayley Scales of Infant Development*[32] that had previously been found for full-term infants. This finding provides an empirical justification for the use of this scale with preterm infants.

3. Internal Consistency of the Instrument

In assessing the internal attributes of a test it is helpful to examine the relationship of subscales and items to the total score. This is especially important when the new test instrument has many components. If a subtest or item has a very low correlation with the total score, the test developer must question the subtest's contribution to the total score. This technique would be most useful in providing confirmation of the validity of a homogeneous test. A test which measures broad groupings of constructs would not be expected to have a high degree of internal consistency.

Bruininks has reported internal consistency research for the BOTMP.[25] He presents comparisons of item scores with subtest and total scores, hypothesizing that an item should be more closely related to its subtest score, a homogeneous comparison, than with the total score which contains more heterogeneous behaviors. His hypothesis was confirmed since all comparisons yielded stronger relationships between items and subtests than between items and total score.

4. Correlations with Other Tests

High correlations with other tests that purport to measure the same constructs, and low correlations with measures that are designed to measure attributes other than the one under study, are further evidence of construct validity. *Convergent validity* is indicated by relatively strong relationships between the developing test and other measures. *Discriminant validity* is indicated by relatively poor relationships between the developing test and measures designed to assess some other construct.[29]

If the new test is strongly related to the performance domain that it was intended to be related to, but also shows a strong relationship to areas that it was not intended to tap, the test would seem to be tapping many factors, including irrelevant ones. In some instances such results could be understood given the type of test task. For example, complex tasks which draw upon a variety of postural, sensory, motor, and higher cognitive functions would be expected to correlate with many different performance measures.

Correlations with other tests are difficult to interpret. If a test has a perfect correlation with another test, then others will question whether the new test is necessary. A perfect correlation means that either test would suffice to answer the same questions. If, however, a test has some unique components to it, one would expect it to produce moderate correlations with another test, indicating that the two are not measuring identical constructs.

As part of test development and validation of the K-ABC, the manual reports correlations obtained with several other criterion measures. Some of the relationships are reported in the section on concurrent validity, since the goal was to measure the relationship between two tests. However, some tests are widely accepted as measures of "intelligence" including the *Stanford-Binet Intelligence Scale,*[33] *Wechsler Preschool and Primary Scale of Intelligence,*[12] and the *Wechsler Intelligence Scale for Children-Revised* (WISC-R)[23] Therefore the correlations between these intelligence scales and the K-ABC are reported in the construct validity section, since the studies were used to confirm the construct of intelligence. These studies are reported in detail in the examiner's manual,[30] but in general many of the correlations are between .70 and .80 depending on the age and exact test being administered. The correlations were relatively high, but not so high as to indicate that the tests are measuring exactly the same construct.

Convergent and discriminant validity studies help sharpen the meaning and interpretation of reported constructs. For more detailed information on convergent and discriminant validity see Thorndike[29] and Anastasi.[28]

5. Differences Between Groups

If two groups with known characteristics can be identified and assessed by the new test, and if a significant difference between the performance of the two groups is found, then incisive evidence of test validity will be provided. The interpretive manual of the K-ABC[30] features an extensive section describing studies which validated the use of the test to differentiate the following groups from normals: gifted and talented, educable mentally retarded, culturally different Native Americans, hearing impaired, learning disabled, dyslexic, trainable mentally retarded, high risk preschool, and behaviorally disordered.

If evidence can be accumulated which demonstrates that the new test discriminates between normals and the group it was designed to measure, the underlying theory is further substantiated and construct validity enhanced.

SUMMARY AND RECOMMENDATIONS

In occupational and physical therapy, the global focus on human performance, an advantage in treatment settings, becomes a liability in instrument development if not carefully managed. Measurement must focus on specific functions or processes, rather than overall performance.

In the therapies, many variables previously have not been studied. This lack of precedents makes validity research difficult. For example, since there are no well-established, standardized measures of postural integrity, if a test developer designs a measure of postural integrity there will be no other tests with which to establish concurrent validity. This does not mean that a new instrument cannot be validated; rather it suggests that the validation process is different than it might be for more generally accepted constructs. For example, the test developer might compare the new test to other clinical judgments, or expert decisions about status to establish the validity of test results.

As new tests are designed to assess performance deficits, a clearer picture of the constructs of interest will become available. Also, the prevailing theoretical conceptions of constructs may evolve and change as a result of ongoing research on the validity of specific tests. The relationship between a validity study and the constructs being studied is a circular one: the constructs are dependent on research findings and research findings clarify the constructs. The ongoing validation process will make possible a fuller integration of theory, research, and practice.

REFERENCES

1. American Psychological Association: *Standards for Educational and Psychological Testing.* Washington, DC, American Psychological Association, 1985.

2. Fisher AG, Wietlisbach SE, Wilbarger JL: Adult performance on three tests of equilibrium, *Am J Occup Ther* 42:30-35, 1988.

3. Campbell DT, Stanley JC: *Experimental and Quasi-Experimental Designs for Research.* Chicago, Rand McNally & Co, 1966.

4. Fuchs D, Fuchs LS, Benowitz S, Barringer K: Norm-referenced tests: Are they valid for use with handicapped students? *Except child* 54: 263-271, 1987.

5. Moore GW: *Developing and Evaluating Educational Research,* Boston, Little Brown & Co., 1983.

6. Payton O: *Research: The Validation of Clinical Practice.* Philadelphia, FA Davis, 1980.

7. American Psychological Association: *Standards for Educational and Psychological Tests.* Washington, DC, American Psychological Association, 1974.

8. Gardner MF: *Test of Visual-Perceptual Skills (Non-Motor).* Seattle, Special Child Publications, 1982.

9. Beery KE: *Revised Administration, Scoring, and Teaching Manual for the Developmental Test of Visual-Motor Integration,* Cleveland, Modern Curriculum Press, 1982.

10. Thurstone LL, Thurstone TG: *SRA Primary Mental Abilities Test.* Chicago, Science Research Associates, 1962.

11. Miller LJ: *Miller Assessment for Preschoolers.* San Antonio, TX, Psychological Corporation, 1988, 1982.

12. Wechsler D: *Wechsler Preschool and Primary Scale of Intelligence.* New York, Psychological Corporation, 1967.

13. Kirk SA, McCarthy JJ, Kirk WD: *Illinois Test of Psycholinguistic Abilities,* Urbana, University of Illinois Press, 1968.

14. Ayres AJ: *Southern California Sensory Integration Test Battery.* Los Angeles, Western Psychological Services, 1980.

15. Frankenburg W. Dodds J, Fandal A, Kazuk E, Cohrs M: *Denver Developmental Screening Test-Revised.* Denver, Ladoca, 1975.

16. Stangler SR, Huber CJ, Routh DK: *Screening Growth and Development of Preschool Children: A Guide for Test Selection.* New York, McGraw-Hill Book Co, 1980.

17. Lieberman S, Cohen AH, Stolzberg M, Ritty JM: Validation study of the New York State Optometric Association (NYSOA) Vision Screening Battery. *Am J Optometry Physiological Optics* 62(3): 165-168, 1985.

18. Lichtenstein R, Ireton J: *Preschool Screening: Identifying Young children with Developmental and Educational Problems.* New York. Grune & Stratton Inc, 1984.

19. Lichtenstein R: Comparative validity of two preschool screening tests: Correlational and classificational approaches. *J of Learn Dis* 14: 68-72, 1981.

20. Meehl P, Rosen A: Antecedent probability and the efficiency of psychometric signs, patterns, or cutting scores. *Psychological Bulletin* 52: 195-215, 1955.

21. Elllison PH: The relationship of motor and cognitive function in infancy, preschool and early school years. *J Clin Child Psychol* 1: 81-90, 1983.

22. Keppel G: *Design and Analysis: A Researcher's Handbook*, ed 2. Englewood Cliffs, NJ, Prentice-Hall, 1982.

23. Wechsler D: *Wechsler Intelligence Scale for Children-Revised*. New York, Psychological Corporation, 1974.

24. Woodcock RW, Johnson MB: *Woodcock-Johnson Psychoeducational Battery*. Hinghan, MA, Teaching Resources Corporation, 1978.

25. Bruininks RH: *Bruininks-Oseretsky Test of Motor Proficiency Examiner's Manual*. Circle Pines, MN: American Guidance Service, 1978.

26. Harris DB: *Goodenough-Harris Drawing Test Manual*. Los Angeles, Western Psychological Services, 1963.

27. Borg WR, Gall MD: *Educational Research: An Introduction*, ed 4. New York, Longman, 1983.

28. Anastasi A: *Psychological Testing*, ed 5. New York, Macmillan, 1982.

29. Thorndike RL: *Applied Psychometrics*. Boston, Houghton Mifflin Co, 1982.

30. Kaufman AS, Kaufman NL: *Kaufman Assessment Battery for Children: Interpretive Manual*. Circle Pines, MN, American Guidance Service, 1983.

31. Meisels SJ, Cross DR, Plunkett JW: Use of the Bayley Infant Behavior Record with preterm and full-term infants. *Dev Psychol* 23: 475-482, 1987.

32. Bayley N: *Bayley Scales of Infant Development*. New York, Psychological Corporation, 1969.

33. Thorndike RL. Hagen EP, Sattler JM: *Stanford-Binet Intelligence Scale*, ed 4. Chicago, Riverside Publishing Co, 1986.

KEY POINTS

1. Validity refers to the extent to which a test measures what it purports to measure. It includes the appropriateness, meaningfulness, and usefulness of the test.

2. Valid and effective test use is directly related to the tester's expertise. With experience the tester becomes better able to evaluate a wide range of problems.

3. Validation of tests involves a series of formal and systematic studies which provide a basis for the interpretation of test

results and evidence that is acceptable to professionals in other fields.

4. Validity is initially investigated as an instrument is being developed, and confirmed through subsequent use. The process is a continuous one which consists of replication and cross-validation. It is accumulated knowledge that cannot be obtained from one study.

5. The test developer is responsible for providing potential users with adequate information to judge whether the test is appropriate for specific purposes and for a targeted clinical population. Cautions about inappropriate use of the test instrument also must be provided.

6. Cross-validation studies are needed to rule out systematic sources of error that may influence test results for different diagnostic subgroups.

7. Content validity is the degree to which test items represent the performance domain the test is intended to measure. Content validity can be established through expert judgments, adequate descriptions of test content and uses, and the development of a Table of Specifications. It is not indicated by a statistical measure, but rather is inferred from judgments.

8. Criterion-referenced validity may be demonstrated by concurrent studies correlating two or more measures, and predictive studies comparing initial test results to later performance on criterion measures.

9. Predictive validity methodology has traditionally been based on correlational methodology but evolved towards classification analysis which allows for calculation of true and false negatives and positives.

10. Construct validity is the extent to which the test is shown to measure theoretical constructs or traits.

11. Construct validity is originated in the planning phase and executed in the development of the test. The methodology used in all aspects of developing and standardizing a test impacts on its construct validity.

12. Major areas to be considered in the validation of constructs include: age differentiation, factor analytic study, internal con-

sistency of the instrument, correlational evidence, and differences between groups.

13. If it can be shown that test scores demonstrate a progressive increase corresponding to age, this will add to the construct validity of tests for children.
14. Factor analysis can assist in determining whether there are several theoretical domains within the same test. It simplifies the test items by grouping common traits.
15. The relationship between subscales and items with the total score helps assess the internal consistency of the homogeneous tests.
16. High correlations with other tests purporting to measure the same construct, and low correlations with measures purporting to measure different constructs are evidence of convergent and discriminant validity respectively.
17. Evidence which demonstrates that the new test discriminates between normals and the group it was designed to measure provides further evidence of construct validity.

Chapter 8

Preparing the Examiner's Manual

Tracy A. Sprong

An optimist is a man who starts a crossword puzzle with a
fountain pen.

—Anonymous

INTRODUCTION ·

The examiner's manual is the focal point of a test. It embodies
critical information regarding the test's purpose, intended uses, theoretical background, qualifications of examiners, technical characteristics, and standardized procedures for administration, scoring,
and interpretation. The manual functions as a learning tool and continual reference for users. Most importantly, it serves as the basis
for evaluation by qualified users of the test's content, technical adequacy, and appropriateness. Test reviews are often based exclu-
sively on the manual, and do not necessarily imply that the reviewer
has administered the test. In essence, the manual reflects the test's
quality.

A manual should be evaluated on the basis of its completeness,
accuracy, and clarity. If the typical user of the manual is likely
to gain an inaccurate impression, the manual is poorly written
. . . Test developers and publishers should, therefore, provide

Tracy A. Sprong, MEd, is Research Assistant with the Foundation for Knowledge in Development, 8101 E. Prentice Ave., Englewood, CO 8101 and a free-
lance technical writer in Denver.

information in manuals to help reduce the likelihood of misunderstanding or misuse of test scores.[1,p35]

The purpose of this chapter is to present a framework and basic guidelines for converting test development research into a useful and adequate manual. Content is based upon a review of 20 standardized test manuals and a variety of technical/scientific writing publications.

PRELIMINARY PREPARATION

Organizational Systems

The manual will be much easier to construct if an organizational system is implemented early on in the test development process. A good system includes specific procedures for collecting information and record keeping. An organized approach can save the researcher hours of time sorting and deciphering notes recorded on scraps of paper and re-checking references at the library. The individual system should reflect techniques with which the researcher feels most experienced and comfortable.[2]

For those writing by hand, Mullins[3] suggests using a notebook with dividers, a large folder with pockets, or a large file box with dividers if writing on index cards. For all methods, she recommends writing the title of each section on the divider.

For those writing by computer, suggestions include: regularly printing out copies, maintaining a key of filenames and brief abstracts of the information in each file, and setting a regular time to enter information from library and field research. Whether using hard or floppy disks, it is essential to make backup copies on a regular basis.

Suggestions for both the hand or computer methods include: noting the date on all drafts; using colors to code and organize information; and setting up a regular "housekeeping" schedule to update information and transcribe notes, bring references up to date, and discard outdated drafts.

References

It is important to be meticulous in recording complete and accurate references *on an ongoing basis* and filing them in a card box or entering them on a regular schedule into the computer. Cox and West[2] suggest that reference cards be grouped by subject which helps writers to be organized and resultant writing easier to follow. Noting where references were located (library, colleague's office, etc.) is helpful in case future re-checking is necessary. Recording full bibliographical information at the time it is collected can prevent frustrating hours in the library re-looking up references. Common details overlooked in recording references include: authors of a chapter in an edited book, volume numbers of journals and books, and page numbers of an article or a chapter in an edited book.

Notetaking Tips

When taking notes from literature sources, it is useful to record the page number of the information (even though it may not be quoted) in case it is necessary to return to the reference.

Keeping a file of definitions, encountered during library research, is helpful for later use in composing the manual's operational definitions or glossary.

When it is too time-consuming to summarize the information on cards or in notebooks, the researcher should obtain copies of relevant papers, articles, chapters, etc.[2]

It is essential for the test developer to maintain meticulous and step-by-step records of the research methodology including information regarding: the sample (selection procedures, size, characteristics), data gathering, reliability and validity studies, and data analysis procedures.

GETTING STARTED

"The major block to writing is the initial step."[4,p225] Writing is an individual process, and different techniques all have advantages and disadvantages. Regardless of the test developer's writing method, it often helps to break up the writing into smaller, more manageable pieces to avoid getting bogged down by the entire task. Outlined below are some workable techniques for getting started suggested by Mullins.[3]

1. Some well-organized authors begin by outlining in detail from beginning to end.
2. Some authors prefer to write from beginning to end with only a rough idea of major sections. A detailed outline is formulated later to review the content and sections which have too much or too little information.
3. Some authors write in bits and pieces, beginning with what they know best and find easiest, then an outline is prepared. This method can help overcome the hurdle for some of getting started.

Audience

Before beginning to write, it is critical to determine who the audience will be. It might be helpful to make a list of anticipated users and their academic and clinical background. It follows that the presentation of information will vary depending upon whether users will be paraprofessionals, college students, practicing clinicians, and/or educators.

The manual will need to be "user friendly," easy to read and understand by the audience targeted. Factors affecting readability are difficulty of vocabulary, length of sentences, complexity of concepts, degree to which the test is specialized, page format, illustrations, writing style, and organization.[3] As Mullins[3] remarked, some of the best writing is done by those who have confidence to write simply and directly.

THE DRAFTING PROCESS

The first draft is written to bring together the bits and pieces you collected throughout the period of the research or over the year(s) as the project developed, to get the essential facts together, to have something to build on, to eliminate nonessentials, and to discover what to emphasize.[5,p12]

The first draft is an opportunity to "brainstorm" and write without worrying about form and style. It is also helpful to put aside the completed first draft for a few days, or weeks before beginning a second draft. The writer can usually catch omissions, irrelevancies, and abruptness by putting the manuscript aside and rereading it later.[6]

After revisions and rewriting, the second draft can then be critically examined for focus, style, grammar, sentence order, etc.[6] Once again, it is beneficial to put the writing aside for a while. It is also worthwhile to read the draft aloud to uncover problems of abruptness.[6]

Another critical phase of the writing process is to ask a colleague to critique a draft. Criticism can be used to stimulate thinking and improve writing.[3] A colleague may uncover many problems with writing or presentation that are not immediately seen because the author has lost some objectivity after having spent so much time with the material.[6]

Mullins[3] suggests that colleagues be chosen for their substantive, theoretical, or methodological competence on the topic; frankness; and reputation for prompt, thoughtful responses. Further, a colleague with a different orientation can be a valuable critic to test the breadth of communication. Specifically, criticism should be requested on the manual organization, content, grammatical correctness, brevity, and writing style. A copy editor should also review a final draft so that the style and flow of the manual will provide clarity and promote efficient use of the test.

In summary, the test developer should be prepared for numerous drafts. As Richardson[5] points out, the art of successful writing lies in revision.

Writing Style

Manuals are examples of scientific writing, a style which is simple, direct and unbiased in tone. "Unconstrained wordiness lapses into embellishment and literary elegance, which are clearly inappropriate in scientific style."[6,p34] General style considerations in scientific writing are noted below.

1. Effective writing is characterized by the use of no more words than is necessary to discuss the topic thoroughly but efficiently.[3,6] Writers tend to become redundant in an effort to be emphatic.[6]
2. Varying sentence length helps readers maintain interest and comprehension. Writing only in short, simple sentences creates tedious reading while long, involved sentences can impede the ready grasp of ideas.[6]
3. Consistent advice given in style and writing guides is to avoid jargon,[3,5,6] the use of a technical vocabulary even in places where it is not relevant. ". . . jargon also grates on the reader, encumbers the communication of information, and often takes up space unnecessarily."[6,p33]
4. "Use adjectives and adverbs sparingly. Some such as *very* and *quite* both weaken and lengthen sentences."[3,p99]
5. It is advisable to carefully examine each sentence and paragraph for ambiguity.[5]

Tables and Figures

Tables are employed when information can be expressed or displayed more clearly and economically than in the text. Information presented in tables should amplify or supplement the text, not duplicate it.[5] A well-constructed table ". . . enables the reader to quickly see patterns and relationships of the data not readily discernible in the text."[6,p83] The *Publication Manual of the American Psychological Association*[6] recommends the following considerations in constructing tables:

1. Rounded-off values may demonstrate patterns more distinctly than precise values.
2. Readers can more easily compare numbers down a column than across a row.
3. The reader can inspect data more easily if a visual focus is provided of column and row averages.
4. Ample spacing can improve a table because white space creates a perceptual order to the data.
5. Tables should be given brief yet clear and explanatory titles.

6. Consistency in the presentation of all tables facilitates comparison within the text.
7. Tables are central components of the text but should be intelligible without references to the text.
8. The unit of measurement or the number of decimal places should be maintained within a column.
9. "An author's thoughtful preparation makes the difference between a table that confuses and one that informs the reader."[6,p84]

Illustrations other than tables are called figures (photographs, graphs, drawings, etc.). Figures should be of professional quality with sharp detail for reproduction. Photographs should be sharp with a contrasting background, and drawings should be made with black india ink on a good grade of bright white paper.[5,6]

FINAL ORGANIZATION

The American Psychological Association (APA) has published a useful guide to the test developer entitled *Standards for Educational and Psychological Testing*.[1] The publication is intended as a technical guide for evaluating testing practices and determining the merit of a test, and elaborates standards regarding the construction and publication of test manuals/user's guides. Standards categorized as "primary," which should be met by all tests before their operational use include: thorough descriptions of the rationale of the test, recommended uses, and cautions against misuses; statements of special qualifications required to administer and interpret the test; and specific information about communicating test results to people who lack the training required to interpret them.

Manual Content

Content areas or "chapters" frequently found in test manuals are elaborated below as guidelines for structuring important information that users will need to evaluate and administer the test. These provisional chapters can be combined or rearranged depending upon the logical order of the material and the intended uses of the test and accompanying manual.

Manuals do not necessarily infer length. Some good manuals are brief, with topics combined and elaborated in a few paragraphs. As with content, length will vary depending upon the purpose of the manual, and essential information and background needed to use the test. For instance, the theoretical background section of the *Carrow Elicited Language Inventory*[7] is summarized briefly for targeted users who are presumed to have specialized training in speech and language.

Some test manuals contain all information in one volume such as the *Miller Assessment for Preschoolers*,[8] and the *Developmental Test of Visual-Motor Integration*.[9] Other manuals are constructed in two volumes, one for administration and scoring instructions and one with technical and interpretive information such as the *Kaufman Assessment Battery for Children*,[10,11] *Comprehensive Identification Process*,[12,13] and *Goodenough-Harris Drawing Test*.[14,15]

The purpose of the *Acknowledgments* section is to recognize those colleagues, organizations, key staff members, and funding agencies that have made contributions to the work. It is important to maintain a professional tone in enumerating their specific contributions. Some test developers include acknowledgments in a *Preface* or *Foreword* which also serves as an introduction to the goals of the test and an overview of the manual's chapter structure.

Chapter 1, Description of the Test, commonly includes: a general description of the test, why it was developed, uses and limitations of the instrument, abilities assessed, and examiner qualifications.

Chapter 2, Administration and Scoring Instructions:

The directions for test administration should be presented with sufficient clarity and emphasis so that it is possible to approximate for others the administrative conditions under which the norms and the data on reliability and validity were obtained ... The directions presented to a test taker should be detailed enough so that test takers can respond to a task in the manner that the test developer intends.[1,p29]

Specific guidelines to keep in mind when writing instructions incorporate the following points:

a. A simple, step-by-step manner is best used to structure directions.
b. The test developer should specify if directions or wording are to be used exactly or are provided as flexible guidelines.
c. Users will need to know of problems or situations discovered during pretest and standardization studies, that can influence test performance.
d. The test developer should anticipate that users will interpret directions differently. It many be necessary to supplement instructions with operational definitions or a glossary.
e. Drawings and photographs can be used effectively to augment directions that are awkward to describe.
f. It is beneficial to adhere to a consistent way of phrasing directions to avoid user confusion, even though it may seem tedious reading. The test developer needs to choose between, for example, "Examiner places card on table to the left of client's midline" or "Place card on table to the left of patient's midline." Labels for a test taker are also more easily understood if stated consistently (e.g., client, patient, child, or individual).

Chapter 2 should include the following: general testing guidelines, item sequence, materials and/or equipment, description of the testing room and setup, and specific directions for administering and scoring each item.

This chapter also includes an explanation of determining the final score. The methods to calculate test performance and instructions in using norm tables are provided. As with administration instructions, scoring procedures are best communicated in simple, step-by-step directions. Norm tables need to be placed in a logical, and easily referenced location. To facilitate accurate interpretation, the test manual should also specify the rationale for the method of reporting scores, and how scaled scores are derived from raw scores.[1]

Chapter 3, Interpretation, provides users with guidance to formulate inferences from item, subtest, and total score performance. Conclusions or generalizations should be reserved for the populations from which the standardization sample was drawn.[16] The presentation of case histories can be a valuable interpretive aid for users. This chapter is also the appropriate location to elaborate potential limitations of the research, cautions in interpretation of test results, and suggestions for future investigation or replication studies. Any use of the test with special populations should also be elaborated in this chapter.

Chapter 4, Theoretical Background, is based upon a review of pertinent literature. This chapter is an opportunity to present users with a sound theoretical or conceptual framework which guided development and supports the purpose of the test. The underlying constructs upon which the validity research will rely should be carefully delineated.

Chapter 5, History of Test Development, details the process through which the test was constructed. It includes: development of initial test items, pilot or tryout testing, description of the Development Edition, procedures for standardization, and development of scoring criteria. In this section, the rationale and supportive evidence are presented of the procedures used in selecting and/or constructing items during the pilot studies and Development Edition. Domain definitions and test specifications are also clearly described so that knowledgeable experts can judge the relationship of the items to the domain they represent.[1]

This chapter generally includes a complete description of the standardization sample. In order for a user to evaluate a test for appropriateness, the manual should include the year in which data were collected, descriptive statistics, and a detailed description of the sampling design and participation rates.[1]

Critical factors in describing the sample include exact size, subgroup sizes, sample selection procedures (random or volunteer), and proportions of the sample by stratification variables (e.g., community size, racial/ethnic group, education, occupation, and income). It is helpful to the user if the characteristics of the population from which the sample was derived are described (e.g., applicable demographic variables of the United States, state, city, or region). A detailed description of pilot study samples, preceding standardization, is also valuable information.

Chapter 6, Psychometric Properties, provides users with enough information to determine if the test's technical characteristics are acceptable for their intended uses and interpretations. This chapter is likely to include extensive tabular material. For the convenience of users, it is preferable to place tables and figures within the corresponding text, rather than at the end of a chapter or in the appendix. Topics commonly addressed in a presentation of technical information are briefly discussed below.

Reliability

In describing reliability studies, the samples should be fully described including the number of cases, selection methods, and their representativeness. In addition, information needs to be provided regarding time intervals over which data were collected and statistical analysis used. "Reporting standard errors, confidence intervals, or other measures of imprecision of estimates is also helpful. Reporting a reliability coefficient alone, which typically varies more from one group of test takers to another, is less informative."[1,p20] The types of reliability studies that were conducted will vary depending on the purpose for the test. However test manuals typically include some or all of the following types' of reliability studies: interrater, test-retest, internal, and standard error of measurement.

Validity

According to APA,[1] a rationale should be provided to support the mix of validity evidence presented (e.g., content, criterion-referenced, and/or construct). Samples need to be fully described including the number of cases (and reasons for eliminating any cases), selection methods, and the representativeness of the sample. Criterion measures and rationale for inclusion should be accurately described. Pertinent information in describing validity studies also includes: time intervals over which data were collected, statistical analysis used, and qualifications of raters or subject matter experts.

SUMMARY AND RECOMMENDATIONS

If contemplating the manual as a whole, the task can seem overwhelming. With careful planning, however, each section can be written during the corresponding phase of the test development process so that by the end of the standardization study, a draft is ready for final editing and subsequent publication. Also, by writing during the development process, the test developer can set his/her own schedule and, to some extent, avoid the pressure of trying to write the entire manual facing the pressure of publication deadlines. Quality efforts rarely result when writing occurs at an unnaturally rushed pace.

Information gathered during the review of the literature, to formulate the test concept and find potential items, will compose the basis of the manual's theoretical background chapter. In full detail, this information can be written into a paper for submission to an appropriate professional, refereed journal with a readership of intended test users. In this way, the test developer can extrapolate information for the manual from a larger, well-written effort that has gone through a process of peer review for content and writing style. Documentation of the item selection process and results of pilot testing, during the Development Edition phases, can provide the basis for another paper submission. This information will be detailed in the manual's history chapter.

During the development and standardization phases, project examiners will provide invaluable feedback on the clarity of administration and scoring instructions. It is likely that this section of the manual will be almost completed before standardization begins. Project testers are also a good source of case studies for the interpretive section.

It is advisable to build writing activities into project timelines and budgets. In particular, statistical and/or test and measurement consultants are good sources of writers and editors for the manual sections on reliability, validity, determining the final score, and interpretation. Content and bias review experts, in the standardization and Development Edition phases, can also be valuable contributors to these chapters.

Theoretical background, item selection, and results of Development Edition studies, well written early in the test development process, can also serve as a basis for funding proposals for further Development Edition and standardization studies. The submission and publication of papers during the development process is also viewed favorably by funding agencies and documents an acceptance within the field of preliminary efforts.

Other test manuals, regardless of their subject matter, are some of the best resources for writing and structuring the manual. While conducting library research or reviewing tests for potential items, it is convenient to make notes on writing style and organization. This process can produce two benefits: what to avoid and what to replicate. The preparation of the examiner's manual is a component of test development and as such, requires the same attention to planning and detail as all other phases of the process. The years of hard work that are involved in the development of a norm-referenced standardized test merit a clearly written, well-organized and comprehensive examiner's manual to reflect the quality of the test.

REFERENCES

1. American Psychological Association: *Standards for Educational and Psychological Testing*. Washington, DC, APA, 1985.

2. Cox RC, West WL: *Fundamentals of Research for Health Professionals*. Laurel, MD, Ramsco Publishing, 1982.

3. Mullins, CJ: *A Guide to Writing and Publishing in the Social and Behavioral Sciences*. Malabar, FL, Robert E, Krieger Publishing, 1983.

4. Stein, F: *Anatomy of Research in Allied Health*. New York, John Wiley & Sons, 1976.

5. Richardson FR: *Author's Style Guide to The American Journal of Occupational Therapy*. Rockville, MD, American Occupational Therapy Association, 1979.

6. American Psychological Association: *Publication Manual of the American Psychological Association*, ed. 3. Washington, DC, APA, 1983.

7. Carrow E: *Carrow Elicited Language Inventory*. Allen, TX, DLM Teaching Resources, 1974.

8. Miller LJ: *Miller Assessment for Preschoolers*. San Antonio, TX, Psychological Corporation, 1988, 1982.

9. Beery KE: *Administration, Scoring, and Teaching Manual for the Developmental Test of Visual-Motor Integration*, rev ed. Cleveland, Modern Curriculum Press, 1982.

10. Kaufman AS, Kaufman NL: *Kaufman Assessment Battery for Children: Interpretive Manual*. Circle Pines, MN, American Guidance Service, 1983.

11. Kaufman AS, Kaufman NL: *Kaufman Assessment Battery for Children: Administration and Scoring Manual*. Circle Pines, MN, American Guidance Service, 1983.

12. Zehrbach RR: *Comprehensive Identification Process: Interviewer's Manual*. Bensenville, IL, Scholastic Testing Service Inc, 1975.

13. Zehrbach RR: *Comprehensive Identification Process: Technical Report*. Bensenville, IL, Scholastic Testing Service Inc, 1985.

14. Harris DB: *Goodenough-Harris Drawing Test Manual*. Los Angeles, Western Psychological Services, 1963.

15. Harris DB: *Children's Figure Drawings as Measures of Intellectual Maturity: A Revision and Extension of the Goodenough Draw-a-Man Test.* New York, Harcourt Brace World Inc, 1963.

16. Isaac S, Michael WB: *Handbook in Research and Evaluation.* San Diego, CA EdITS Publishers, 1981.

KEY POINTS

1. The manual embodies critical information regarding the test's purpose, intended uses, theoretical background, qualifications of examiners, technical characteristics, and standardized procedures for administration, scoring, and interpretation.

2. The manual will be easier to construct if an organizational system is implemented early on in the test development process. A good system includes specific procedures for collecting information and record keeping.

3. It is important to be meticulous in recording complete and accurate references on an ongoing basis. Noting where references were located is helpful in case future re-checking is necessary.

4. To make writing the manual easier, the test developer should maintain meticulous and step-by-step records of the research methodology and procedures.

5. It often helps to break up writing the manual into smaller, more manageable pieces to avoid getting bogged down by the entire task.

6. Before beginning to write, it is critical to determine who the audience will be. It might be helpful to make a list of anticipated users and their academic and clinical background. The presentation of information will vary depending upon the intended users.

7 A critical phase of the writing process is to ask a colleague to critique a draft. Criticism can be used to stimulate thinking and improve writing.

8. Writing style tips include: use of as few words as possible, varying sentence length, avoidance of jargon, spare use of adjectives and adverbs, and careful examination of each sentence and paragraph for ambiguity.

9. Tables are employed when information can be expressed more clearly and economically than in the text. Information pre-

sented in tables should amplify or supplement the text, not duplicate it.

10. It is preferable that figures reflect professional quality preparation with sharp detail for reproduction.

11. Manual length will vary depending upon the purpose of the manual, and essential information and background needed to use the test.

12. Manuals can be constructed in an all-inclusive manner or in two volumes, one for administration and scoring instructions and one for technical information.

13. For the convenience of users, it is preferable to place tables and figures within the corresponding text, rather than at the end of a chapter or in the appendix.

14. Directions for test administration should be presented clearly and in enough detail so users can approximate the conditions under which the norms and the data on reliability and validity were obtained.

15. Administration and scoring instructions are best communicated in simple, step-by-step directions.

16. A meaningful approach in presenting interpretation information is to reserve conclusions or generalizations to the populations from which they were drawn.

17. In order for a user to evaluate a test for appropriateness, reports of normative studies should include the year in which data were collected, descriptive statistics, and a detailed description of the sampling design and participation rates.

18. Domain definitions and test specifications should be clearly stated so that knowledgeable experts can judge the relationship of the items to the domain they represent (test validity).

19. Reliability and validity studies should be accurately described. Test developers should consider postponing publication of their test manuals until sufficient reliability and validity data are accumulated so that test users can determine the value of and best uses for the test.

20. Other test manuals are some of the best resources for writing and structuring the manual.

Epilogue

Test Development
on the Installment Plan
or
"How I Developed a Test
in 27,000 Easy Steps"

"Begin at the beginning" the King said gravely, "and go until you come to the end; then stop."

Lewis Carroll
Alice's Adventures in Wonderland *(1865)*

Whenever I present a workshop on the MAP (Miller Assessment for Preschoolers), someone always asks, "Why did you become a test developer?" It seems like such an odd question, like when I was growing up I would have decided that I wanted to become a Developer of Tests. That isn't the way it happened. As I begin to answer, I hear a familiar tape recording begin . . .

In the early 1970s I was working in the Head Start program in Boston. As part of my job (which also included working in the clinical nursery school program, and being an occupational therapist on the infant stimulation team) I was responsible for screening the children in the Boston Head Start program. There were 5,000 children in that program!!! Being a new graduate (from the basic master's program at Boston University) and being young, daunt-

Lucy Jane Miller, PhD, OTR, is the developer of the *Miller Assessment for Preschoolers* and Executive Director of the Foundation for Knowledge in Development, 8101 E. Prentice Ave., Englewood, CO 80111.

less, and perhaps foolish (?), I embarked along a path from which I have found it impossible to turn.

I began to test the children in the Head Start program, and tested, and tested! At that time the only available screening test was the *Denver Developmental Screening Test* (DDST).[1] As the weeks turned into months, and then into years it became glaringly apparent that the DDST was "missing" many of the children with a variety of problems, later identified by teachers. I then began to develop a simple checklist which I used in addition to the DDST in evaluating the abilities of these preschool children. (There are hundreds, maybe thousands, of this kind of criterion-referenced checklist in existence. Probably everyone reading this has developed one at some time.)

Luckily (I think) Massachusetts in 1975 passed a law similar to Public Law 94-142 requiring that all preschoolers be screened and treated if identified with problems. At that time, the checklist I had constructed and called the "Developmental Screening for Pre-schoolers" (DSP) was in its infancy, but had been used for several years in the Boston Head Start program. Several of the school systems in the surrounding area heard about the checklist, and contacted me to see if I could train their staff to administer it.

Even though I knew next to nothing about research and data analysis, I knew it was supposed to be done. I was hesitant to see the DSP checklist in widespread use, because no data on it had been gathered in a systematic fashion. Finally, after many hours of negotiations, we decided that the school systems could use the DSP checklist if they signed a contract which acknowledged that it was in the Development Phase, and I, in return, could use the data obtained from testing the children in each school system.

This was in the days before computers (not before they were invented, but before I had enough courage to face one). Thus analyzing the data from the children who had been tested involved taking my calculator (I wasn't afraid of those) and calculating average scores on each item for each age group. I had heard of Buros' *Mental Measurements Yearbook*[2] in graduate school, thanks to Pat Wood's class, and I went to the library and began to read all the reviews that had been written about any tests developed for children. I began what later became one of my infamous lists, which noted (by test) all of the criticisms that were made in Buros about tests for children. (It was a long list.) I decided that I did not want my test to have any of those problems. So I started to develop my test by learning all the things not to do!!

I had been exposed to the early work of Dr. A. Jean Ayres in a class taught by Sharon Cermak. I was stimulated and intrigued. So I called Dr. Ayres and said, "I am a graduate student at B.U. and I am really interested in doing a traineeship with you for the summer. I would be happy to pay for the privilege." (I still can't believe I had the courage to do that. Calling famous people makes me nervous.) To my astonishment, she said yes and I began one of the most stimulating experiences of my professional life.

Dr. Ayres taught me much more than the theory of sensory integration. She taught me to be a critical thinker, an asker of questions. She helped me to question everything *she* was doing, and by implication, everything I was doing.

When I returned to Boston, I realized I would have to obtain funds to continue my work (I wasn't comfortable calling it research yet). At that time I changed jobs and became the head of a preschool program for emotionally disturbed children. (Work on the test was still on an evenings, weekends, and vacations basis.) Luckily for me, Wendy Coster was also on the staff. With my "right" brain, and her "left" brain, we began to write grants to get some funding for the development of the test. The first grant we received was for $500.00 from the Sargent Dudly Allen Fund of Boston University, and it seemed that we had won the lottery. The funds were used to get all the data that had been gathered so far keypunched, and ready for analysis. (I was still afraid of data analysis, but by now I knew about statistics consultants.)

For two years I remained in this job and tried to save as much money as possible to use on hiring consultants to help me keypunch and analyze the data that was obtained testing the public school samples. During this period I was lucky to be in a training program where everyone was trained and supervised in the art of psychotherapy with young children. What I learned from Judy Singer, Louise Wylan, and Joann Fineman shed a completely different perspective on evaluating young children, and convinced me not to give up.

Finally, my husband and I sat down for what had become an

institution in our family, the "Now what?" discussion. We decided that I had to either continue to work, or continue to develop the test, but that I couldn't continue to do both. So we set an arbitrary deadline of two years to get "big" funding. Funding was necessary to implement a national Development Edition, and Standardization Edition of the preschool test. (By now I had come to realize that too many OTs and PTs were unable to complete quality research because they were relying on volunteer samples, volunteer examiners, volunteer statisticians . . . volunteer everything. I *vowed* to pay for the services of the testers and staff on the project.)

I searched for funding by trial and error. I frequented the public library where there was a Foundation Center with reference books on available funding, and read everything I could find on the subject. Several publications suggested that prospective grantees conduct interviews with the agencies to which they were applying prior to submitting applications, to assess the appropriateness of the project for the funding institution. Therefore I began a series of sojourns to Washington to meet with Directors in BEH, MCH, NIMH, NIH, etc. (I am fond of saying that any agency that ended with an "H," I visited!)

I brought with me (besides persistence) a one-page description of the project, and a one-page summary of the proposed budget. I received lots of excellent information about applying for funding. I learned that in every agency there is someone whose job it is to meet with prospective applicants and honestly try to help them. It was an invaluable experience.

Then, with Wendy Coster's help, I began to apply for funding. It was a depressing and difficult process. A grant proposal typically took two to three months to write. Then there was a several month waiting period (during which another grant would be written) and then generally a letter saying that the grant proposal was turned down.

During this period, I received a real boost through a grant awarded by the American Occupational Therapy Foundation (AOTF). This award allowed me to pilot test items nationwide using volunteer therapists to collect initial data. Although the reliability of the data gathered was questionable, the award was invaluable, because in subsequent grant applications, I could demonstrate previous support, and some data.

Finally, only weeks from the end of my self-imposed two-year deadline, I received word that a grant I had submitted under the auspices of AOTF had been ranked first on scientific merit. However, because it was our first grant, there was an enormous amount of "red tape" to fight through before the funding could be approved. Thanks to the strength and cunning of Wilma West and others, these hurdles were overcome and we began our project.

We had been funded to field test a Development Edition and a Standardization Edition of the test nationwide. It was a one-year grant. Thus we had three months to construct the Development Edition and kits, three months to field test it, three months to analyze the data and construct the Standardization Edition and kits, and three months to administer the Standardization Edition. Many, many lessons were learned "the hard way" during this phase. There were numerous excellent consultants who assisted with item content and training the examiners such as Lana Warren (in the area of neurodevelopment). There were also several extreme disappointments such as a tester who lied about having tested her sample, and did not admit that she had no children tested until two weeks before the end of the project. (During those final two weeks six examiners were trained and with the help of Pamela Lemerand, Charlotte Royeen and others in that geographic location, 130 children were randomly selected and tested!)

At the end of the year with the help of 12 dedicated, overworked and underpaid occupational therapist Field Supervisors, and a wonderful Research Assistant, Alice Finn, we had accomplished all that we said we would in the grant. We had administered and analyzed the Development Edition, and administered the Standardization Edition. I had all the raw data but no test!! Time for a "Now what?" discussion.

Along the way, the KID Foundation (Foundation for Knowledge in Development, a 501 (c)-3 private nonprofit foundation) had been set up to protect the copyright to the test. The KID Foundation approached several publishers at that time, but they were not interested in publishing a standardized but nonexistent test by an unknown author.

Finally I decided to take out a bank loan to "finish up" the work on the MAP. (By this time the test had become the MAP, thanks to creative thinking by my husband, and me overcoming some misguided humility about use of my name in the title.)

This decision heralded in a new era. With the brilliant assistance of Dick Cox, the scoring system was finalized. I learned how to manage (and mismanage) a small business: how to design, manufacture, assemble, inventory, market, pack, ship, and invoice test kits; and how to pay interest on big loans!! At that time I had a 3,000-square-foot warehouse for an office and spent most of my time struggling through the blue-collar phase of test development!

I learned hard lessons about test materials. At the time I was constructing the MAP, I was interested only in which items had good psychometric data, were fun for children, easy to administer, etc. It never occurred to me to check the cost of materials. If I were to do it all over (and for some reason I think I will with another test), I would carefully consider not including items that require expensive materials, no matter how excellent the psychometric data appears. Why make an excellent test that no one can afford?

I also decided at that time to start the first series of MAP Seminars, to inform people about the test, and to try to repay the loan that had been taken to finish up the development of the scoring system and to manufacture the test kits. I wanted to have experts at the MAP Seminars so that experts in each field would be able to explain their specialty to the participants. I was lucky enough to find wonderful consultants who made the videotape series for me: A. Jean Ayres, Lorna Jean King, Lana Warren, Ann Grady, Judy Singer, Dick Cox, Garie Morgenstern Stein, Allan Eisenbaum and Bill Whalen. A very special Occupational Therapist helped get the seminar series underway, Sharon Murphy Hudgens. In the first two years we held about 30 Seminars.

Time for a "Now what?" discussion. Clearly, I had to get rid of the manufacturing and distributing business if I wanted ever to do research again. And I had a burning desire to find out if the MAP was *accurate* in predicting preschoolers "at risk." Many people told me not to do predictive validity research. They said I was "cutting my own throat" because no preschool test could be predictive after a significant time had passed. But if the MAP wasn't identifying the right children what use was it? I had learned years ago from Dr. Ayres that I had to question the usefulness of the test until proven.

So several things happened. I found a wonderful colleague to help me write grants, Tracy Sprong, who has been with me ever since; I found a small manufacturing firm to take over production of the test kits and signed a five-year contract (that seemed like an eternity at the time); and I decided that if I was going to get into the running for grant funding I would have to have a doctorate, so I got into a PhD program.

One note of gloomy unreality entered at this time. A remarkably negative review of the MAP was published in the *American Journal of Occupational Therapy*. It was devastating, and yet had been published in the main forum of occupational therapy literature. The immediate ramifications of this inaccurate review were catastrophic, including one state not adopting the MAP for use on a state-wide level, and a pending grant not being funded. Two long years later, exemplary reviews were published in Buros' *Ninth Mental Measurement Yearbook*,[3,4] the benchmark publication of test reviews. Reviewers comments included: "In summary, the MAP appears to be the best available screening test for identifying preschool children with moderate 'preacademic problems.' . . . It fills a clear need for professionals working with preschoolers and will quite likely play a major role for many years."[3,p976] ". . . this instrument will take its place along with a handful of others in providing much needed information concerning the learning potentialities of both the so-called normal and learning-disabled preschool child."[4,p978]

For the next several years, I spent uncountable hours applying for grants to complete the predictive validity study. With the assistance of Pamela Lemerand and Tracy Sprong, I was *finally* awarded in 1984 a one-year grant to find as many children as possible from the original standardization sample (who by then were in second, third, and fourth grade) and retest them and examine their records to determine their status. The predictive validity results were remarkable, considering that there had been a *four-year delay* between original testing and the predictive validity study. Now finally I felt that the MAP could be used by therapists and others with reasonable confidence!!

Finishing my doctorate and completing the predictive validity study occurred simultaneously. Time for another "Now what?" talk. It was clear that scraping along from grant to grant was not a satisfactory way to survive. After a very convoluted lucky set of coincidences we finally ended up connected with a man, Pat Pietro, who wanted to set up a series of Thrift Stores, and needed a non-profit to be sponsored. So to make a long story short, the KID Foundation is now the proud owner of two, soon to be three Thrift Stores. We have about 60 employees, and are proud that our stores are the cleanest and nicest in town!!! We hope to someday have a stable financial base for our continuing research endeavors, independent of the vagaries of grant funding.

Meanwhile, I found out that there was funding available for *for-profit* companies, through the Small Business Innovation Research (SBIR) program. So I started another company, Developmental Technologies Inc., a for profit, Research and Development company. After several applications, Developmental Technologies was awarded an SBIR Phase I grant to pilot a short form of the MAP. Currently our Phase II grant has been submitted, and we are waiting with crossed fingers to hear the results. If funded, we will be in business for two years! The first year will be running the Development Edition of the MAP-Screen nationwide, and the second year will be Standardizing the MAP-Screen. The plan is to use this seed money to start a test development company for occupational and physical therapists.

In addition, I have recently been awarded a grant from the American Occupational Therapy Foundation to begin work on an item pool for a new test, the Miller Infant and Toddler Test (MITT). (The AOTF grants always seem to come when I feel like giving up. They keep me going. This year I have had 10 grants turned down, each of which took approximately two months to write.) The new infant and toddler test will be structured according to the new Public Law 99-457 and will have items in each of the five areas required to be assessed by that law: motor, language, cognitive, behavior and self-help. Through the generous funding provided by AOTF, pilot versions of the motor items are currently being field tested, and items are being developed in each of the other four domains. We plan to develop a screening as well as a diagnostic form of this test.

Other ideas are percolating as well: a test for gifted and talented, an activity program for infants and preschoolers, a screening for learning disabilities in school-age children, normative studies for Spanish-speaking children, normative studies for Native American children, normative studies for other ethnic and socioeconomic minorities, translations and standardizations in other countries (already underway in Japan, Israel, Denmark, Canada, Brazil), a school for preschoolers . . . just to name a few.

I spend about 80% of my time trying to find funding to complete the projects I design. My idea of heaven is a place where there is enough money to create the reality of a test, without having to waste time trying to get money to do the project!!

One truly remarkable event has occurred within the last few months. The contract with the small manufacturer was coming to a close (I can't believe it's been five years already!), so we again queried potential publishers regarding publication of the MAP. The Psychological Corporation, through Bob Zachary, responded and the MAP is being published by them as of February, 1988. This is a remarkable validation of the test, and hopefully will help position and legitimize psychometric testing within the field of the therapies.

Why did I become a test developer? I didn't start out to be one. I don't have a special interest in statistics, only children. I like to ask questions, and I want to know the answers. I don't give up easily. And most of all I have had lots of luck and infinite support from family and friends.

Why did I spearhead a project to write this book? Partially because I get so much correspondence from therapists which begins, "Dear Dr. Miller, I have an idea . . . and I just don't know where to go from here." If I had had this volume as a how-to manual when I developed the MAP, it would have made my task considerably easier. I would like this volume to make your job considerably easier. I know you are out there; and I know you just need a little encouragement to begin to formalize your checklist into a norm-referenced tool. Don't be afraid to start at the beginning!! No one ever got to the end before they started.

In 10 years, I would like to edit another collection which is entitled "A Review of Twenty Five Norm-Referenced Tests by Occupational and Physical Therapists." If we combine the research and theoretical expertise of our academic scholars with the amazing energy and enthusiasm of our clinical workforce, what we can accomplish will astound everyone, even ourselves. I did it; we can do it; *YOU can do it.*

Lucy Jane Miller
Who became a test developer
April, 1988

P.S. It is essential that a test developer have a strong support system because it can be a lonely and demanding job. In preceding drafts of this epilogue I closed by thanking the people who have supported me at those times when I felt like giving up. However since the list of names took up a page and a half, I had to omit them from the manuscript. You Know Who You Are . . . I thank you all.

REFERENCES

1. Frankenburg WK, Dodds JB, Fandal AW, Kazuk E, Cohrs M: *Denver Developmental Screening Test, Reference Manual,* rev ed. Denver, CO, LaDoca, 1975.

2. *The Mental Measurements Yearbook.* Lincoln, NE, Buros Institute of Mental Measurements, University of Nebraska, 1985.

3. Deloria DJ: Review of Miller Assessment for Preschoolers, in Mitchell JV (ed): *The Ninth Mental Measurements Yearbook.* Lincoln, NE, Buros Institute of Mental Measurements, University of Nebraska, 1985, pp 975-976.

4. Michael WB: Review of Miller Assessment for Preschoolers, in Mitchell JV (ed): *The Ninth Mental Measurements Yearbook.* Lincoln, NE, Buros Institute of Mental Measurements, University of Nebraska, 1985, pp 976-978.

Appendixes

APPENDIX A

CRITIQUE FORM FOR NORM-REFERENCED STANDARDIZED TESTS

Category

BASIC TEST INFORMATION

	Yes	No	NR*	Comments
Clear descriptions provided of purpose and need for test.				
Examiner qualifications and training described.				
Time required to administer test provided.				
Age group test intended for detailed.				
Administration procedures detailed so user can approximate standardization conditions.				
Item format and response format suitable for test purpose and intended users.				
Manual written in style appropriate for intended users.				
Test materials appropriate.				
Additional materials provided by examiners fully described.				
Cost of test and scoring materials reasonable.				

SCORING AND INTERPRETATION

	Yes	No	NR*	Comments
Scoring materials well-designed and easy to use.				
Scoring criteria are clear and well-defined.				
User can easily convert raw scores to final scores.				
Confidence bands can be determined for test scores.				
Tables in easily referenced location for users.				
Guidelines provided for interpreting and communicating scores.				
Limitations of scoring system described.				
Appropriate cautions noted regarding:				
Size of the sample				
Population from which sample drawn				
Use of test with other populations				

* Not Reported

197

Category

DEVELOPMENT PROCESS

	Yes	No	NR*	Comments
Rationale for test purpose described.				
Pilot research and Development Edition studies well-described:				
sample number and characteristics				
sample selection procedures				
test-retest reliability studies				
interrater reliability studies				
validity studies				
Item analysis conducted including:				
item discrimination				
item difficulty				
intercorrelations between items				
quality of item distractors (when appropriate)				
other				
Oversampled subgroups to check for item bias.				
Review panel involved to analyze ethnic and gender bias.				

STANDARDIZATION PROCESS

Standardization sample well described:

sample number and characteristics

sample selection procedures

random or stratified random sampling plan used

characteristics approximate intended population

Yes	No	NR*	Comments

* No Reported

Category

	Yes	No	NR*	Comments
STANDARDIZATION PROCESS (Continued)				
Item analysis conducted including:				
item discrimination				
item difficulty				
factor loading				
bias analysis				
other				
Reliability				
Administration and scoring procedures objective.				
Reliability examiners and training described.				
Reliability samples adequately described.				
Reliability samples representative of the population for which test intended.				

Rationale provided for selecting types of reliability studies.

Test-retest reliability reported and within acceptable range.

Interrater reliability reported and within acceptable range.

Internal consistency reported and within acceptable range.

Reliability is reported for:

    each age level

    each subtest

    total test

Validity

Research methods and measures well-described and easily replicable for further cross-validation.

Validity examiners and training described.

Validity samples adequately described.

* Not Reported

201

Category

STANDARDIZATION PROCESS (Continued)

Validity

	Yes	No	NR*	Comments
Validity samples representative of the population for which test intended.				
Rationale provided for selecting types of validity studied.				
Evidence of content validity reported:				
expert judgments procedures specified				
test content and uses related to objectives				
Table of Specifications well-constructed				
other				
Evidence of criterion-referenced validity reported:				
Criterion measures described and rationale provided for selection.				
Concurrent data in an acceptable range.				

Predictive validity:

classification analysis in acceptable range

correlational analysis in acceptable range

Construct validity described and in an acceptable range:

age differentiation

factor analysis

internal consistency

correlational evidence with other tests

differences between normals and specified subgroups

constructs upon which test is based are
operationally defined

other

* Not Reported

203

APPENDIX B
DIRECTORY OF SELECTED TEST PUBLISHERS

Academic Therapy Publications
20 Commercial Boulevard
Novato, CA 94947-6191
(415) 883-3314

American Guidance Service
Publisher's Building, P.O. Box 99
Circle Pines, MN 55014-1796
(800) 328-2560

Childcraft Education Corporation
20 Kilmer Road
P.O. Box 3081
Edison, NJ 08818-3081
(800) 631-5652

Children's Hospital of San Francisco
Publications Dept.
P.O. Box 3805
San Francisco, CA 94119
(415) 750-6165

Common Market Press
P.O. Box 45628
Dallas, TX 74245
(214) 247-5945

Consulting Psychologists Press, Inc.
577 College Avenue
P.O. Box 60070
Palo Alto, CA 94306
(415) 857-1444

Cornell University Press
P.O. Box 250
Ithaca, NY 14851
(607) 277-2211

CTB/McGraw-Hill
Del Monte Research Park
2500 Garden Road
Monterey, CA 93940
(800) 538-9547

DLM Teaching Resources
P.O. Box 4000
One DLM Park
Allen, TX 75002
(800) 527-4747

Educational Testing Service
Rosedale Road
Princeton, NJ 08541
(609) 921-9000

Grune & Stratton, Inc.
111 Fifth Avenue
New York, NY 10003
(407) 345-4200

Jastak Associates, Inc.
1526 Gilpin Avenue
Wilmington, DE 19806
(800) 221-9728

Charles E. Merrill Publishing
  Company
1300 Alum Creek Drive
Box 508
Columbus, OH 43216
(614) 258-8441

Modern Curriculum Press
13900 Prospect Road
Cleveland, OH 44136
(800) 321-3106

Pro-Ed
5341 Industrial Oak Boulevard
Austin, TX 78735
(512) 892-3142

Psychological Assessment
  Resources, Inc.
P.O. Box 98
Odessa, FL 33556
(813) 977-3395

The Psychological Corporation
555 Academic Court
San Antonio, TX 78204-0952
(800) 228-0752

The Riverside Publishing Company
8420 Bryn Mawr Avenue
Chicago, IL 60631
800-323-9540

Scholastic Testing Service, Inc.
480 Meyer Road
P.O. Box 1056
Bensenville, IL 60106
(312) 766-7150

Science Research Associates, Inc.
155 North Wacker Drive

Chicago, IL 60606
(312) 904-7000

Special Child Publications
P.O. Box 33548
Seattle, WA 98133
(206) 771-5711

Stoelting Company
1350 South Kostner Avenue
Chicago, IL 60623
(312) 522-4500

Western Psychological Service
12031 Wilshire Boulevard
Los Angeles, CA 90025
(213) 478-2061

Printed and bound by CPI Group (UK) Ltd, Croydon, CR0 4YY

17/10/2024

01775688-0001